P9-CLE-027

The Answer
to Cancer

The Answer to Cancer

IS NEVER GIVING IT A CHANCE TO START

ℬ

Hari Sharma, M.D. and
Rama K. Mishra, G.A.M.S.
with James G. Meade, Ph.D.

SelectBooks, Inc.

The Answer to Cancer
© 2002 by Hari Sharma, Rama K. Mishra and James G. Meade.
All rights reserved.

This edition published by SelectBooks, Inc. For information address
SelectBooks, Inc., New York, New York.

All rights reserved. Published in the United States of America.
No part of this book may be used or reproduced in any manner
whatsoever without the written permission of the publisher.

First Edition

ISBN 1-59079-018-9

Manufactured in the United States of America

10 9 8 7 6 5

❦ Dedication

To His Holiness Maharishi Mahesh Yogi

❧ Acknowledgments

We want to thank Maharishi Mahesh Yogi for bringing out the Vedic knowledge in a very simplified and understandable way, making it available to anyone. Because of the understanding he has brought, we have been able to bring out the simple health techniques and suggestions in this book.

We also want to acknowledge all of our families for their patience and support during this ambitious undertaking. Thanks to Dr. Manohar Palakurthi for his helpful suggestions, and thanks to Nick Sharma, Ellen Kauffman, and Surya Kant for their beneficial editorial assistance. We also want to thank our publisher, SelectBooks, and its heads—Kenzi Sugihara and Bill Gladstone—for all they have done.

Disclaimer

This book is not a "miracle cure" book for cancer, and we don't recommend that you use it in that way. If you have been diagnosed with cancer, see a physician and follow his or her advice. This book is prevention. Does fastening your seat belt guarantee that you won't be a traffic fatality? No, but it's still a good idea, and it saves lots of lives. Our suggestions in this book are a "safety belt" for averting cancer. They're effective, but the book makes no other claims.

� Contents

✌ Introduction

This is a short book. You've probably noticed that already as you hold this modest stack of pages in your hand. Nothing to it. Yet, the book is confronting *the* most perplexing, traumatizing, miserable, mean, unsolvable sickness of all time. Even big books haven't been able to address the matter with much success. Libraries of books. How can this little book do it?

Well, being little is part of our point. Cancer happens at the tiniest level of the body—at the level of the cell and the cell chemistry. But that's not why we've made this book little. This book is little because it's the simple things that work—simple things, but things our modern civilization has gotten away from. We thought that a simple book would be the best way to convey our message that you should do the simple things (like eat veggies).

So the book is short. Still, sometimes it helps right at the outset to know how the book works and how you can get the most out of it (while doing the least). So right at the beginning, we'll explain a few things.

Who Ought to Read This

When you call something a "cancer book," that immediately suggests that the book is directed at people who already have cancer. To be honest, it's a bit of a "spin" problem for us, because we actually want to reach another, more considerable portion of the population—namely, all those who don't have cancer yet.

The suggestions in these pages certainly are useful for those who have already encountered the ugly disease. Those with cancer benefit if they start right now doing the things they should have done to prevent cancer from coming up in the first place. We also have in mind those who have previously had it, and folks in that category may indeed be motivated to ask, "What can I do so that this doesn't happen again?" We can mention, too, that these techniques are good for a lot more than cancer prevention; they can be used to simply promote health.

Our intended reader is the everyday person who does not yet have cancer and is in the enviable position of being able to prevent it from ever arising. Some people know that the threat of cancer is considerable. A mother, brother, sister, or cousin may have developed the sickness, and such people may feel that they are at risk. We certainly have these people in mind for this book. Likewise, those with moderate risk may be our audience—such as those who have reached the age where, statistically, their chances of falling sick from cancer seem to increase.

There is no one who has absolutely no risk of getting cancer, so there is no one we do not have in mind as we prepare these pages. And that, above all, is our point. We're thinking of the everyday person as we make these recommendations—the relatively healthy person driving to work, going to college, mowing the lawn, watching soaps on TV, dining out, or, in general, living in the mainstream of life without that much concern about their health.

The thing is, we want people to start making a few, simple adjustments to their routines right now, before they get sick, so that they won't ever get cancer. The whole approach may be a lot less macho than waiting until people develop cancerous tumors and then trying to expunge the spreading malaise. Yet, it's an approach that really works…much more effective than if you wait until the disease appears.

The character of our audience helps to explain a couple of things about this book—first, it's shortness, which makes sense when we're trying to appeal to those who aren't that eager to learn about these materials anyway; second, it's tone, which we discuss a bit in the next section.

Why the Lighthearted Tone

Cancer books tend to be somber. If you scan the table of contents here, you'll see that this book isn't somber. It's light, playful, and easy. Why have we done that? We intend no disrespect. First of all, you don't necessarily help someone who feels worried if you act worried yourself. A little humor does much more than sobriety to cut the tension. Our main reason for the lighthearted tone is to entice people into reading our simple suggestions.

Face it. At least some of the information in here is available elsewhere. Some of the secrets from the *Vedic* tradition you won't find in Western scientific texts. But you could probably find much of it somewhere, even in other books by the authors. Maybe you could find some of this material in the scientific literature. But would you read it if you did find it? What are the numbers here? How many people ever read the average scientific article? A hundred? We're aiming at something more like a billion. We want people to know these things, and that's why we're holding ourselves to high standards of offhandedness, relaxation, and easiness. Information doesn't have to be hard-to-get to be good.

Also, we want to assure you that in drawing upon *Vedic medicine,* we take considerable strides to *avoid* classical terminology from Vedic medicine. The terminology is new to most people, and even our colleagues in the medical profession complain that they can quickly get lost in the onslaught of terms that are new to them—body types, channels in the body, specific imbalances. (Have you ever heard of a *shrota* before? It's a channel, but the point is that we avoid that terminology.) A small amount of the terminology creeps in, but a very, very tiny amount. You won't have any trouble with it.

In short, we want you to read these short pages...all of them...and that's why we wrote them the way we did. Besides, as we explain in our chapters on "being nice," light-heartedness is actually a cancer fighter. So the tone of the book is a preventative therapy.

How to Get Under Way (Not Overwhelmed)

Simple as any given suggestion may be in this book, the advice does tend to pile up. This is a *book* after all, not a single paragraph, and we worry about overwhelming you in spite of ourselves.

So here's what to do. Just start with something that appeals to you. Some readers may do many of the recommended practices in here; others may do almost none. Don't feel that you have to do everything in here immediately. Who would even start then?

You might choose to read through the whole book, and we've done our best to make it easy to do that. Or you might skip around. That's OK. As for getting yourself started on these gentle therapies, choose something. Maybe the stewed apple in the morning. Maybe the techniques to cut back on sugar. Maybe improved sleep. When you start with one or two, you'll find yourself easily picking up others as well. There's a momentum to the whole thing. Healthy people seek out healthy habits.

The overall benefit of the practices we recommend is a long, healthy, and happy life. But you shouldn't feel pressured to do everything at once. You can start with maybe some food supplements and just add the diet and lifestyle tips here and there as you go along.

We do have a plan to the book, as you can see from looking at the table of contents. Basically, we go from the most tangible things (like food) to the more abstract things. You can read the book and begin to follow the recommendations in the sequence we provide. But you really don't have to do them in any specific sequence. You might start being nice before you start increasing the phytochemicals in your diet. That's good. You can do these things in any order at all, whatever is best for you.

It's a good idea to keep this book around for, oh, forever or so. After you've been through it, just pick it up again from time to time to remind yourself of things or to find suggestions you'd overlooked. "Oh, here's a good way to use turmeric in a milk shake," you might discover one day, or "So, my body makes anticancer chemicals while I sleep. I think I'll get to bed early tonight." Read the book, enjoy it, get healthy, and browse through it again and again. It's your friend.

Who Are These Authors?

Western medicine has credibility, particularly with Western people. Vedic medicine has thousands of years of tradition and credibility with non-Western people. Not wanting to leave either direction uncovered, this book is a blending of East and West, as are its authors.

Hari Sharma, M.D., the lead author, might sound like he's from India, and he did start out there. But he is a full-fledged Western physician. He was Director, Cancer Prevention and Natural Products Research, Department of Pathology, College of Medicine and Public Health, The Ohio State University, Columbus, Ohio[1] (yes, the university with the great football team). He is now Professor Emeritus. He's published more than 120 research articles and written three other books so far, listed in the Reference section at the end of this book. One, *Freedom from Disease,* reflects his ongoing determination to make people healthy. Another book he co-authored, *Contemporary Ayurveda,* shows that he is an expert in Vedic medicine as well as Western medicine, and he loves to bring the ancient practices into the modern world. He has lectured worldwide on his research and *Ayurveda.*

1. Institutional endorsement not implied.

Speaking of Ayurveda, the second author—Dr. Rama Kant Mishra—is an Ayurvedic physician, known in India as a *Vaidya*. He is a Graduate of Ayurvedic Medicine and Surgery (GAMS), from SYNA Ayurvedic College, Bhagulpur. He has spent plenty of time in the West, and is a distinguished member of the Council of Maharishi Ayurveda Physicians. He has been in private practice since 1974 and knows how to work with people to make them healthier. (Dr. Sharma is also in private practice.)

So the authors know the modern, Western way. They know the ancient, Eastern way. And they know how to bring them together to help real people. They just thought they would package all that know-how in a book that people would read. They came to the third author, Jim Meade, Ph.D., to help them to do that. Dr. Meade, whose Ph.D. is in English literature, has written 23 previous books...some of them in the funny and quite famous *Dummies* series.

Mixing West and East

There is some Western science in here. There is some *Veda*, too (Veda, which is a somewhat new term for our non-Eastern readers, means total knowledge for the evolution of life, and refers to the ancient, mainly oral tradition preserved over the millennia in India.) What is the place for each?

The Western science is to satisfy the mind of the reader—you know, your mind. Tell somebody to eat leafy vegetables because they are nutritious and enrich the body, and that somebody kind of shrugs. "What are you talking about?" Tell him or her that the leafies have beta-carotene, lutein, and folate; and their intellects begin to be satisfied. It's just the way we are in our world. If we know the scientific explanation, we begin to accept things. If we don't, the whole subject may be just "folk wisdom" to us, and we won't eat our leafies. When there's a scientific explanation, backed up by hardcore research at respected institutions, we say, "Fine. Pass the spinach."

What about the Eastern tradition—the Veda? It takes natural approaches, based on consciousness and consideration of the whole body. Because consciousness exists at even an unseen level and is working all the time in the body, it has wide-ranging effects. Vedic medicine works at that level, with the knowledge of which herbs affect which types of consciousness and where, and when to allow that to happen. Vedic tradition provides the know-how in the book, with the full understanding that the reader won't be inclined to accept it unless the Western verification is there as well.

In this way the book provides both Western science and Vedic science. It's a nice synergy.

Isn't the Title a Bit Exaggerated?

It really isn't. Simple, natural things are the answer to cancer. Getting back to basics will do it. Cancer can only happen when cells get away from their basics. If you don't let that happen, you won't let cancer happen.

But being simple isn't automatic. We've been getting away from basics for a long, long time, and we've forgotten how to get back there. We don't sleep right. We don't eat right. We don't transcend right. And there are simple ways to get back to doing all those things the right way—simple, painless ways that your body and mind appreciate.

But you can't really do it on your own. You need some guidelines. It isn't that simple to be simple. We've done our best to make it easy in this book, and we truly know of no other book like it. As far as Western books go, they usually don't have the understanding of the whole body and how it works. Somebody may rediscover, for instance, that tomatoes are cancer fighters. (Somebody has, in fact.) Then they'll do something along the lines of advising you, "Eat a raw tomato every chance you get. Eat one for breakfast. Have one at bedtime." And they might neglect all the other things you should be doing right along with eating tomatoes. Besides, you might get sick from eating all those tomatoes.

Drawing upon the Vedic tradition, we know the right uses of these fruits and vegetables—the right timing, the right combinations, the right interactions. We make it all sound falling-off-a-log simple. It is. But you still have to know how to do it right, and we tell you how.

There is a short answer to the question of whether or not the title to the book makes excessive claims. "No, it doesn't." The book is a short answer to cancer...an answer with long-term effects. Do these things, and you'll feel great, day after day. You'll just forget about cancer altogether, which is exactly as it should be.

PART ONE

&

Quick Start
"Cancel Cancer"
Techniques

❦ One

The "ABC" of Cancer: A Basic Conundrum

"CANCER." There may be no more terrifying word in our language. "Shark," "tsunami," "tornado," or "incoming" might be other candidates, but they hardly surpass "cancer" in striking fear to the heart.

Though medicine has some success in treating some cancers some of the time, it has very little success in treating all cancers all of the time. Even when it treats them successfully the first time, it does little to prevent them from coming back again. In some cases, such as lung cancer and pancreatic cancer, an unfavorable diagnosis is close to a death sentence.

These depressingly familiar words about killer cancer are nothing new. Here are some other words, almost as familiar as the depressing ones (although few of us seem to be paying attention as they're so frequently said).—"Research has shown that most cancers can be prevented. Scientists now estimate that 60 percent to 70 percent of cancers are preventable through currently available information and simple changes in diet and lifestyle," says the American Institute for Cancer Research on its Web site.

3

"Preventable deadly disease." It almost sounds like an oxymoron. It is the basic conundrum we are addressing. Cancer is preventable, yet people are getting it left and right. Clearly, something is missing, and perhaps that something is quite simple—some diet guidelines, a few herbs, some adjustments to the daily routine, a few insights into the emotions and the mind.

An "answer to cancer" may not be nearly as impossible as modern thinking would have us believe. Perhaps we have simply become habituated to reacting to cancer after we get it instead of taking steps to render it powerless before it ever starts.

A Disease Out of Control

Certainly cancer is continuing to defy all attempts to treat it successfully. And if you go by the numbers, it seems like everybody is at risk for developing cancer. The American Cancer Society says that men in the United States have a 1 in 2 chance of developing this dreaded disease in their lifetime. Women are only slightly better off, with a 1 in 3 chance of falling victim to cancer.

Here are a few more numbers, just to emphasize what everyone knows—that cancer is commonplace and hardly any family escapes its ravages altogether.

There are 8,900,000 Americans alive today who have already had cancer. In the 12 years between 1990 and 2002, doctors diagnosed 16,000,000 cancer cases in the U.S. An estimated 555,000 Americans are expected to die of cancer in 2002—more than 1,500 a day. According to National Institutes of Health estimates, cancer is costing the US $157 billion a year. We know the numbers are pretty mind numbing, but it's good to make clear that we're addressing an epidemic here and not just some minor complaint.

Figures are similar around the world. The United States stood 24th in the world in Death Rates from Cancer per 100,000 population. Hungary ranked number one, France 5, Italy 10, Canada 22, and Australia 25.

For smokers, the American Cancer Society offered these sobering numbers in a 1996 publication:
- Chance of dying in a single airline trip—1 in 815,000.
- Chance of dying in a single skydiving jump—1 in 96,296.
- Chance of being killed in a car accident before his/her 65th birthday—1 in 143.
- Chance that smoking will kill him/her by the age of 65— 1 in 5.

To drive home its point that cancer is relentless and difficult to avoid, the Cancer Society says, "Judging strictly by the statistics, your chance of surviving a shark attack is actually better than your chance of surviving...certain cancers. Worldwide, only seven to ten people die each year from shark attacks." (The Society fails to point out how many people survive shark attacks, but the point is pretty unmistakable. Certain cancers are deadly.)

What are the most common types of cancer? Of the 1,284,900 new cancer cases expected to be diagnosed in 2002 in the U.S., 205,000 are breast cancer, 189,000 are prostate cancer, and 169,400 are lung cancer. Colon cancer accounts for 107,300 and skin cancer accounts for 58,300.

Doctors, by and large, openly admit that medicine is failing in the war against cancer. There's even been a study published in the *New England Journal of Medicine* that reached this conclusion. Here are a couple more such statements from medical professionals, with such admissions being about as hard to find as skyscrapers in Manhattan. "Certainly a new approach to the treatment of cancer was—and still is—desperately needed," observes Candace B. Pert, Ph.D. in her book *Molecules of Emotion.* "Although the cancer establishment has been trying to crack this disease for years," she continues, "it continues to kill more people every year, often a slow and painful death made even more excruciating by toxic treatments."

Dr. Joseph B. Campbell, in a letter to the *Townsend Letter for Doctors* in November, 1994, summarizes the hopeless cycle of Western medicine. "The development of antibiotics, such as penicillin was a great boon to humanity, yet it had some adverse effects. If cancer was caused by an organism, then all we had to do was find another Wonder Drug. Billions of dollars and enormous effort has gone into finding this cancer cure. It has spawned a Cancer Establishment involving many scientists, doctors and a multitude of supportive people. Governments and the general public have been generous in supporting this elusive failed search."

Cancer—Cells Gone Bonkers

What is this disease that is stubbornly defying treatment? Is there something inherent in cancer that makes the disease difficult to prevent, even though we have the tools to do it?

Well, cancer *is* a condition that takes place at a small, complex area of the body—namely the DNA that controls cell functioning—and not on the same gross structural level as a bloody nose or a broken leg.

Cancer, according to the American Cancer Society, "is a group of diseases characterized by uncontrolled growth and spread of abnormal cells." Cancer results when the DNA of the cell—the cell "brain" that regulates all its activity—doesn't work right any more. The cancer cell, you could say, is crazy…a real weirdo at loose in the body.

The DNA-genetic system controls cell reproduction. The DNA also tells the cell what to become, such as a liver cell or a stomach cell. In cancer, the DNA either doesn't send signals, sends wrong signals, or sends signals that the cell ignores.

The healthy cell works as a contributing part of an organ, such as the liver. The cancer cell, with its incorrect signals, "forgets" that it is part of an organism. It may not stop growing when it should. It may not become the type of cell that it is supposed to become.

Clusters of uncontrolled cells form a tumor, and the tumor can damage healthy cells around it by robbing the healthy cells of nutrients and oxygen or by producing harmful chemicals. Cancer cells, in short, are wackos running loose in the body. They forget what they are. All they think about is reproducing themselves (even though they don't know what they are reproducing). They lose all identity and any useful function in the body. And they take over from all the good, useful cells in the body that do know themselves and do perform good work. Nobody likes cancer cells.

Modern Treatment—The Sledgehammer Approach

How is our contemporary, Western medicine approaching this dread killer? In other words, "What are we doing that basically isn't working anyway?" First of all, modern medicine hardly focuses on prevention. It treats cancer primarily after it has shown up as cancer, not before. Second, even though cancer is a disease that originates in the DNA and not the structural level of the body, the treatments work—guess what?—on the gross structural level. Not much of a formula for success.

Take a look at what medicine does—surgery, chemotherapy, and radiation. Surgery, chemotherapy, and radiation. Surgery, chemotherapy, and radiation. If it sounds like some kind of a crude stopgap, that's because it is. Overwhelmed by the disease, medicine attacks the symptoms at the surface, not the cause at the root. What it does is better than nothing, but only slightly. It's hardly an "answer."

Surgery means cutting out the cancerous area. Chemotherapy, rather than addressing a specific area, addresses the whole body. Doctors generally use it for cancers that have spread (metastasized). The theory behind chemotherapy is that drugs can stop those "out of control" cells (cancer cells) from growing or multiplying. Radiation therapy, like surgery, focuses on a specific area that is cancerous. High-energy x-rays or rays from radioactive substances destroy the cells in that area.

These treatments really have almost nothing to do with out-of-control DNA. They don't think of cancer cells as normal cells gone awry; they think of them as foreign invaders and simply try to annihilate them.

Treatment Side Effects—Pain

These modern treatments are pretty violent. You wouldn't choose to have anything to do with them if you felt you had any choice. Surgery doesn't just cut out the cancerous portion of your tissues. To assure getting all the malfunctioning cells, surgery also cuts into your healthy tissues…often into a lot of healthy tissue. In having a tumor removed from a breast, you may also lose a breast, some muscles, perhaps much more. The polite term for what happens in surgery is "side effects," and, as mentioned, you wouldn't go for surgery at all unless you were highly motivated.

Radiation, which burns out the tumor, also burns out more than just the cancer. It burns some healthy tissue. The burns have to heal and are unpleasant. Chemotherapy doesn't just kill cancer cells. It kills some cells that are maybe just a little more vulnerable than others and even some healthy cells. Widely known side effects of chemotherapy can be nausea, vomiting, sores in the mouth, and hair loss. Radiation may cause the same side effects, depending on which part of the body it is treating.

Chemotherapy and radiation also make you susceptible to illnesses, because they weaken your immune system. Even when they're successful, they usually mean that you trade one sickness for another. Some people feel worse from the treatment than from the cancer. There is no point in disguising the truth that some people die from these treatments.

In the ultimate irony, cancer treatments can even cause cancer that you wouldn't have gotten in the first place. Tamoxifen, for instance, is a drug that looks to the body like the female hormone estrogen. It does slow the growth of breast cancer cells, which is good. It can be helpful after surgery in keeping the breast cancer from coming back. However, this estrogen imitator also has some of the harmful effects of estrogen. It increases the risk of cancer of the uterine lining, because it stimulates that lining to grow.

Cancer Causes—Things That Drive Cells Crazy

Might not medicine develop effective treatments if it addressed the causes of cancer? Science can point the finger at a number of causes, both within the body and from the external environment. But for the most part, it does little to address those causes.

Cancer generally develops slowly, over a period of ten years or more, and it can arise not just from a single factor (like smoking) but from a combination of factors (like smoking, alcohol, and diet). Smoking, of course, is the "smoking gun" in all kinds of cancer cases. It's linked to a third of all cancer deaths in the United States. If most people know little about cancer prevention, they at least know that smoking is linked to cancer. Yet many continue to smoke. For the most part, medicine does little more to help people stop smoking than advising people to do so.

If you listen closely, you'll also hear modern medicine saying that diet is a known risk factor. High-fat foods, especially from animal sources, can increase your chances of getting cancer, says the American Cancer Society. Such a high fat diet correlates with cancers of the colon, rectum, prostate, and endometrium (the lining of the womb). Conventional medical sources frequently note that cancer can develop if you eat too many smoked, cured, pickled, or charred foods. Some medical sources are beginning to note the link between sugar and cancer.

Being overweight is a risk factor. Studies have found that people who are more than 40 percent overweight have a much higher risk of developing colon, breast, prostate, gallbladder, ovarian, and uterine cancer. Alcohol increases the chances of getting cancer of the mouth, larynx, throat, and esophagus.

Some of the risk factors for cancer come from within the body. Hormones, immune conditions, and inherited mutations can disrupt the normal functioning of the DNA. The female hormone estrogen, for example, may contribute to breast cancer and other cancers in women. Some cancers appear to run in families, arising from a predisposition to the disease and from inherited mutations.

The environment also poses risks. Though many cast a suspicious eye on pesticides, the American Cancer Society rates them as only an "Unproven Risk." (DDT is a proven carcinogen, and many are equally skeptical of the "safer" chemicals that have replaced it. If these new pesticides wreak havoc on the cells of insects, couldn't they damage our cells as well?)

Chemicals can be carcinogens, with asbestos and arsenic being two good examples. Radiation can cause cancer. With repeated exposure to x-rays, metal detectors, and even just the sun, the DNA of the cell absorbs radiation. The effects are cumulative and can break down the DNA. Electromagnetic fields may cause cancer by disturbing the electromagnetic fields of our body (and breaking down the cell's intelligence).

Science continues to look for underlying causes of cancer. One recent theory is that free radicals in the system contribute to cancer. This theory has the advantage that it does address the very level of the body where cancer seems to develop— namely, the molecular level, where DNA does its work.

Here's a quick explanation of free radicals and cancer. Electrons, to get us started here, are the negatively charged particles around every atom's nucleus. Some oxygen molecules, and other molecules and atoms, are short one of those little particles, which earns those molecules and atoms the name "free radicals." (Depending on your political inclinations, "free radical" might or might not sound like a good thing. In the case of the human body, these marauders mostly aren't good.) Lacking an electron, they attack atoms and molecules that do have enough electrons and try to grab one for themselves. It's a microscopic assault and battery going on in the body all the time. The more free radicals you have, the more assault is going on.

Many of the known causes of cancer also contribute to the growth of free radicals in the body. Smoking, alcohol, and pollution all increase the numbers of free radicals.

Prevention? An Afterthought, At Best

It wouldn't be fair to say that our familiar Western medicine completely disregards prevention as a way to deal with cancer. It would be fair to say that it pretty much disregards it. Beleaguered medicine pays the merest lip service to it while diving wholeheartedly into…surgery, chemotherapy, and radiation.

When medicine speaks of "prevention" it mainly is speaking of early detection, which—if you think about it—isn't cancer prevention at all. It only works when people already have cancer. Early detection may be death prevention, and that's important. But it is not cancer prevention.

Women over 40 are encouraged to have an annual mammogram (to detect breast cancer), and women over 18 are urged to have an annual Pap test (for cancer of the cervix). Men are encouraged to have a prostate-specific antigen (PSA) blood test every year. Both men and women over 50 are urged to get tested for colon and rectum cancer.

Once medicine does detect cancer in an early stage, it turns to…surgery, chemotherapy, and radiation.

If you are motivated and look in the right places you can find anti-cancer recommendations from modern medicine. You've no doubt heard some of these:

- Don't smoke
- Be moderate in drinking alcohol
- Eat fruits, vegetables, and whole grains
- Avoid high-fat foods, especially from animal sources

You may even see a cute poster on the wall of your doctor's office telling you to eat fruits and vegetables. You could just as easily miss such advice altogether. Medicine puts its weight behind treatment. The National Institutes of Health estimate that direct medical costs total $56 billion. Over half of those direct costs are for treatment of breast, lung, and prostate cancer. Little if any of that expenditure is for getting people to eat apples, oranges, and cabbage—foods that medicine well knows are helpful in preventing any number of sicknesses, including cancer.

Here is a summary of our situation at present, then (with a few notable exceptions, such as this book):

First, cancer is enjoying a great boom, devastating as that is to the human population. It's running amok in society, much as cancer cells run amok in the body.

Second, medicine knows what causes cancer—a breakdown in the DNA. But it doesn't work on DNA to solve the problem. It knows many of the causes, but it doesn't do much to address them either. Perhaps it is simply too overwhelmed by the need for instant, gross solutions to the existing problem, such as surgery, to be able to look for something gentle and indirect— like apples for people who don't even have cancer.

Third, prevention really, really does work. Medicine knows that. The most trusted sources like the American Cancer Society even say that prevention works in some startlingly high percentage of cases…such as 60 percent. The percentage could even be much higher. It could be 90 percent. The authors of this book don't rule out that prevention could work on 100 percent of cancers.

Would it be inappropriate to suggest that perhaps all of us looking for an answer to cancer might turn our attention in another direction? Instead of bludgeoning the raging disease, when the condition has all kinds of force and is truly hard to handle, mightn't we make adjustments to the human body so that DNA doesn't go bad and cells don't go berserk in the first place?

Our answer to cancer is as simple as that—to nourish the cells of healthy people so that cancer doesn't come up, much as loving, stable homes nourish children and decrease the like-lihood that the children from those homes will run amok on society.

Unlike surgery, radiation, and chemotherapy, the approaches we discuss in the following chapters *do* work on the level of DNA and—we may as well tell you right now—even at deeper levels than that, at the level of emotions and at the level of the consciousness of the cell that structures the DNA.

These approaches can turn undeveloped cancer into a helpless pretender, a hapless nothing. They can make it irrele-vant. Yet they are so gentle and natural that, if you do them, you won't even think of yourself as treating a disease. You just won't get sick.

❧ Two

Start with a Sassy Stewed Apple

A *stewed apple? A stewed apple in the morning, first thing?* We're talking about a virulent killer (cancer) normally treated with chemicals whose names you can't pronounce and have never heard of, such as—Cyclophosphamide (Cytoxan), Methotrexate, 5-Fluorouracil (5-FU) and Doxorubicin (Adriamycin).

Those unpronouncibles sound potent. But…apples?

"You're going to stand there and tell me that step one in your 'answer to cancer' is a *stewed apple* in the morning? Do you want to lose all your credibility before you even open your lips? A stewed apple? Why don't I just wear my socks backwards? Or wear a potato around my neck? Or how about dance a little jig every time I step out my front door, twirl my finger in the air, and wink?"

If these words don't describe your exact feelings as you embark on this chapter, they may nevertheless approximate what you're thinking. A stewed apple in the morning to treat cancer?

Well, yes, that's what we're saying. It's not the whole program, and it's not really to treat cancer but to prevent it. But, basically, yes, we're putting an awful lot of emphasis on a little red-skinned piece of fruit (and you don't even eat the skin). A 10-ounce stewed apple (or stewed pear, if you prefer) every morning will really bolster your cancer defenses. But it has to be stewed. You have to do it early in the morning. You should do it almost every morning. Let's look at this suggested health step more closely.

A Reason to Bother: Land and Seed Theory

A basis for adopting the stewed apple approach and other rec-ommendations in this book is a simple theory—the land and seed theory.

Cancer seems to strike at random these days. Anybody can get it—any age, any occupation, any personality. Kind, loving people seem to get it almost as much as mean people. Cancer strikes the rich as well as the poor. Cancer may at times seem to strike one geographical area more than another, but it strikes all areas. Pleasant farmers are at risk because of the farm chemicals they've been using for generations. Run to the city and you're at risk from air pollution. Some families seem to have a predisposition to the disease, but the other families usually end up with cancer victims of their own. This disease seems to be indiscriminate and utterly inscrutable. Could there be a simple answer?

Certainly it would be difficult to attempt to address every one of the causes from within and outside the body. However, Ayurveda (the ancient medical practice at the heart of the pre-vention in this book) provides a theory that might encourage all of us to take heart in the face of the seemingly ever-present danger of cancer.

"If you're strong enough, cancer doesn't stand a chance," the theory goes. The name of this traditional theory is "land and seed theory," and what it says is, "The body is the 'land' and all the cancer-causing baddies are the 'seed.' If the land is infer-tile, no matter how strong the seed is, it won't grow." Normally,

16

nobody wants to be infertile. However, in this theory infertility is good.

Traditional Ayurveda says that you can get your body to be so strong that no matter what "germ" comes along—including cancer—you won't get sick.

According to the theory, if the environment is particularly bad, you have to be particularly strong (i.e. infertile) to make up for it. If a seed is strong and the land is infertile, yet the environment is supportive to cancer, well then the disease might stand a chance. You want to minimize your environmental risks if you can. (For instance, don't smoke.)

The worst situation is where the seed is good (i.e. cancer risks are high, with perhaps many free radicals), the land is fertile (your body doesn't have strong immunity to sickness), and the environment is supportive of the disease (maybe you're living on top of a toxic waste dump). In that worst of all possible "land and seed" conditions, well, yes, cancer can happen.

The good part is that you can turn this theory to advantage. Create a body that "just says no" to sickness—a strong body with a strong immune system; a pure, healthy, balanced body. Minimize the risks from your environment as well. Create such a fortress that you don't have to worry about cancer even if it does attempt to invade. Or, according to the land and seed analogy, create a body that is totally inhospitable to cancer, and you won't get it. The seed will fall on infertile land and simply be of no consequence at all.

Ayurveda offers a prescription that helps to create "infertile land"—a body where cancer will find no encouragement and will simply get nowhere. A step in that prescription is a stewed apple to begin the day. Now we're not saying that this one prescription in itself is the only thing you need to do to prevent cancer. There are a lot of chapters in this book, and they all contain good approaches to preventing cancer. We're saying that the apple is a good start. It's easy. Anybody can do it. It costs about a dime a day—basically, nothing. We're putting this technique at the beginning so you can begin to experience success right away.

Science, the Apple, and Your Good Start

Thanks to all the mighty breakthroughs Western medicine has made in fighting everything from bubonic plague to whooping cough, we tend to have confidence in any approach for which Western science offers its support. We're disappointed to confess that we don't have complete support from Western science for our stewed apple recommendation. To our knowledge, no one has done a comprehensive, controlled, longitudinal study of the stewed apple in the morning and its anti-cancer effects.

However, hardly anyone is likely to see any harm in the idea of taking a warm apple to start the day. To give at least some credibility for the Western reader, here are some of the ways Western medicine suggests that a stewed apple may be healthful for you. (Later in the chapter, we tell of some of the Ayurvedic secrets that more fully expose the true power of the deceptively unassuming morning apple.)

Filled with Good Fiber

Fiber. The health world loves it. For something that is basically inert, fiber has become the absolute darling of health circles. And, yes, apples have fiber—lots of it, and it's the good kind.

Apples are rich in pectin, which is a soluble fiber. In fact, apples have more pectin than any other fruit. Perhaps this is enough to clear up any doubts about the morning apple.

Apples also have insoluble fiber, and medicine is well aware that the soluble and insoluble fibers help to clean out the intestinal tract. In other words, fiber bulks up your stool (a polite word for excrement) and speeds the path to elimination for your body's wastes. "Taking out the garbage" is really good for the body, and good for preventing cancer.

It's obvious why fiber might be good for preventing colon

cancer: the less time odious substances spend lying around in your colon, the less time they have to disrupt cell functioning and create confused, dangerous, blind, self-serving cells (i.e. cancer).

Fiber does other good things:

- It helps keep blood sugar and insulin at a steady level. (Sugar, as we explain in a later chapter, can be a carcinogen, too.)
- Fiber helps keep your appetite satisfied. If your gut feels full, you don't feel the need for a couple of candy bars. (Overeating and obesity can contribute to cancer.)
- Fiber stimulates the body to produce substances that regulate the growth of cells in the colon lining. (Regulated growth is good. It's unregulated growth that happens during cancer.)
- Fiber collects and holds bile acids. Acids just running loose can wreak havoc of their own, even if they are good for digestion. Soaking them in fiber and letting them out a little at a time is a nice way to get their good effects without the bad.
- Soluble fiber helps to lower cholesterol, better known for its link to heart disease but also something that just may feed cancer as well. Cholesterol clogs things up, and clogged things can stagnate. Things that stagnate can begin to lose their normal functioning. (We think you see where this is heading.)

As the American Institute for Cancer Research says in a summary, "Fiber dilutes harmful substances, speeds their elimination—and prevents constipation in the process."

Armed with Flavonoids

Fiber alone might seem enough reason to eat your morning apple, but science contributes other good reasons as well. Researchers have recently been discovering an appealing group of nutrients called flavonoids that help strengthen the body and fight disease. As science becomes more and more

19

familiar with the disease-preventing powers of the flavonoids, those nutrients are earning clinical, scientific, hard-to-remember, impressive names like "Nutraceuticals," "Phytochemicals," "Phytonutrients," "Phytofoods," "Functional foods." These names help us to stop thinking of apples as "just food" (which we don't think has much to do with sickness) and instead think of those same, humble apples as "drugs" which can help the body in all kinds of beneficial ways.

To start with a familiar nutrient, we can note that apples have vitamin C. Now, to be honest, they don't have that *much* Vitamin C—only about 12 mg. (It's only about 10 percent of the recommended daily intake of Vitamin C.) However, they pack the punch of a lot more than their 12 mg. More on that in a moment, when we talk about the antioxidant effect of apples.

Apples also have a pharmaceutical-sounding anti-cancer flavonoid called quercetin. According to the U.S. Apple Association, quercetin has demonstrated an anti-cancer effect (possibly by slowing the effects of estrogen, the female hormone that has been shown to contribute to cancer in some instances).

Boasting Impressive ORAC Value

The flavonoids in apples have been shown to have a high ORAC value. Although the term is beginning to catch hold, very few people actually know what ORAC stands for. So, until we explain a bit more, the ORAC value of apples won't motivate too many people to eat this fruit to start the day.

All right. You ready? ORAC stands for Oxygen Radical Absorbance Capacity. Apples help the body increase its absorbance of oxygen radicals—the potentially cancer-causing free radicals we mentioned in Chapter One. Foods with high ORAC values soak up free radicals and deradicalize them. Free radicals, remember, are atoms or molecules scavenging around for an extra electron. Well, apples can create the situation where the radicals end up with those missing electrons…rendering them harmless.

One study looked at the effect of apple flavonoids on the growth of colon cancer and liver cancer cells in the laboratory. The study found that with these apple phytonutrients around, cancer cells didn't grow as fast as when the flavonoids weren't present.

Two-thirds of a medium apple provided as much of an attack on free radicals as 1,500 mg of vitamin C. Here's how the modest 12 mg of vitamin C in the apple suddenly becomes important. Researchers suspect that the combination of the 12 mg of vitamin C with that pharmaceutical-sounding quercetin creates the Vitamin C effect that is 100 times more than the vitamin C alone (yet all entirely natural, without side effects).

Tickling with Trace Minerals

For an added health kicker, apples have some nice trace minerals in them.

They have potassium, which helps regulate water balance, your levels of acidity, your blood pressure, and your neuro-muscular function. It even plays a role in the electrical impulses transmitted in the heart.

Apples also have boron. Science so far says the health benefits of boron are "largely unexplored," but they do think it's probably good. (One study found that boron may help in keeping the beneficial effects of estrogen during menopause.) Some suggest that it's beneficial against arthritis, and it contributes to healthy bones by helping take calcium into the bone structure.

The Right Way to Eat Your Anti-Cancer Apple

Perhaps, with so much said, you know enough to want to ingest this innocent-looking, yet powerful aid to your successful anti-cancer activity. But, for your stewed apple to work right, you should take it right.

First, stew it. If you eat the apple cold, as an aunt of ours once observed, the apple just sits there like a lump in your stomach. If you stew the apple, it's easier to digest. Your sleepy body gently accepts it without complaint and begins to enjoy its benefit. The stewed apple balances your digestion and your level of energy without creating that lump in your stomach.

Second, take it first thing in the morning. Timing is everything. Suppose, in a worst case scenario, you decided "well, I'm getting up late tomorrow, so I'll get a jump on things and take my stewed apple at night." Bad idea. The day has natural rhythms; the body has natural rhythms. The idea is to attune the one (the body's) to the other (the day's). If you have your stewed apple first thing in the morning, you balance the digestion to start the day. If you have it before bed, you signal your body to start digesting at a time when it should be shutting down.

Third, eat an organic apple. Cancer, remember, is a disease of the DNA or even deeper levels of the cell. When you eat food, it breaks down into fine particles that affect those deeper levels of the cells. You don't want some of those particles to be little bits of toxic material from chemicals farmers use to make their jobs easier.

Fourth, eat a non-genetically-engineered apple. The explanation is the same as for eating an organic apple, though the fine particles involved may be even smaller. A genetically engineered apple may have non-apple genes on its DNA—like fish genes or something. When your body is interacting with quercetin and vitamin C and boron and soluble fiber, you don't want it to be ingesting tiny pieces of fish at the same time. Who knows what those fish genes are going to do? The body won't know either, and may get confused. (Avoiding cancer is all about avoiding confusion.)

Fifth, eat a fresh apple. The point is to get the nutrients from the apple while they're lively. Fresh apples have more nutrients. Fresh, tree-ripened apples are best of all.

Sixth, eat a sweet apple. Sour apples in the morning create some imbalance. They make the body work hard. The point of a stewed apple is to get the body working well without making it work hard. Here is a simple way to prepare your stewed apple:

A Simple Recipe for a Stewed Apple

1. Peel a Red Delicious or Yellow Delicious apple.
2. Cut it into quarters, and remove the core.
3. Pierce the apple with 4 cloves, one in each quarter.
4. Boil the combination in water for about 5 minutes or so, to a nice softness.
5. Once the apple is the way you like it, take out the cloves and throw them away. Their job is done. Sit down, and comfortably enjoy this love-warmed, energy-enhancing fruit.

Sip a nice cup of warm water along with it (purified water is best).

In the mood for a more gourmet approach? Here's another recipe:

A More Elaborate Recipe for a Stewed Apple

Ingredients (for one person):
    1 fresh, sweet apple
    5 whole cloves
    ¼ cup of purified water

Directions:
1. Peel the apple, core it, and dice it into small pieces.
2. Put the apple, the cloves, and the water in a covered saucepan.
3. Stew the apple on low heat for 30–45 minutes, until it gets a mushy consistency.
4. Let the mixture stand for 5 minutes away from heat to cool.
5. Take out the cloves and discard them before serving.

Helpful tip: It is best if you sip a cup of warm water with your apple in the morning.

Reminder: We don't recommend this delightful dish at night. It wakes up your digestion, instead of quieting it down. Always take your stewed apple as breakfast first thing in the morning, as early as possible. Even at sunrise.

The Real Power of the Apple (from Vedic Medicine)

Western science offers some small insights into the anti-cancer power of the stewed apple. But the insights aren't all that much, not really enough to convince you to eat the apple instead of, say, a potato (or nothing at all, as people commonly practice).

Ayurveda, on the other hand, offers some secrets that are quite compelling. The apple doesn't carry the anti-cancer load all by itself. The body is a powerful thing, and the apple, you might say, is a trigger to set off the body's own protective mechanisms.

To be honest, we prefer to avoid technical terms from Ayurveda. Our Western colleagues tell us that the Ayurvedic terminology can be overwhelming. People get drowned in the terminology, and they don't get what we're saying.

So, we plan to limit our Ayurvedic terminology, and to give it out in small doses over the course of the book (sort of like the small apples you might eat each morning over the course of a lifetime).

Nevertheless, three little Sanskrit words from Ayurveda tell this story so well that we can't help using them. They help explain just why a single apple can help unleash the power of your own body so that you become a "land" that is utterly repellent to the cancer "seed." These three terms are *agni, ama,* and *ojas.* So, with our apologies for the unfamiliar terminology duly noted, here we go with explanation that we think will help you see how a little stewing and proper timing transform the Clark Kent apple into a Superman for your body.

Agni

Agni is the digestive fire. (If you want to think of the main digestive agni in Western terms, think of the digestive enzymes.) The little stewed apple is a spark to light the digestive fire of the body. Though the simple Western explanation sees digestion happening basically in the stomach (or in the stomach and a few connected organs), Vedic medicine sees digestion happening throughout the body. There are actually lots of agnis, not just one. The little apple can light them all. Digestive fire creates the kinds of substances in the body that keep cells healthy, and it burns away the kinds of impurities that wrongheaded critters like cancer cells thrive on.

We're being pretty low key about it, because agni isn't a familiar term to Western readers. But agni is quite important, and its Western equivalents show that it is important. This "fire" or "flame" is completely in charge of metabolism (breaking down your food into molecules and energy) and of the endocrine systems (your hormones and all that they do). When your body gets out of whack in some way (too tired, too hot, too cold), your agni goes out of whack. On the other hand, if your agni is not disturbed in any way, you just can't get sick.

This potent fire that we all have in our bodies includes all your digestive enzymes (which digest the food and then get it assimilated into the body). It nicely manages how your cells do their work in the all important digestive organ—the liver. It keeps the liver working right and keeps the right biochemicals flowing there. It works at the level of the cells everywhere in the body, not just in the tissues but even in the spaces between the tissues.

It would be tough to try to manage all these things—digestion, liver cells, all cells, tissues, and the gaps between them. But if you know how to manage agni, you manage one thing that takes care of all those digestive and metabolic considerations.

Ama

When agni is not working well, the body builds up ama (the second Ayurvedic term we can't resist introducing). Ama, though unfamiliar in Western medicine, is the great cancer culprit of all time. It's cancer's support system. It's the degenerate, misguided, sticky stuff that clogs cells, confuses them, and can eventually allow them to turn cancerous.

If you were to take all the "bad stuff" circulating in the body and lump it together with a single name, that would be ama. It's germs. It's partially digested food. It's oxidized LDL (the bad cholesterol). And it's lots more bad things, circulating not just in your blood vessels but at the tiniest levels of the cell. It may be a by-product of free radical damage in the physiology.

Not convinced yet? We don't blame you. You need more to go on. Let's take another look at ama from the hard-nosed, Western perspective. Ama is all the accumulated toxins in the body—one name for all the bad stuff you wish wouldn't be there. It's not just a name. It's a real substance. If you don't digest your food fully because of poor digestion or overeating or even irregular daily routine, what do you get? Ama. Forgive us for using the term "slime," but ama is a thick, slimy substance that goes all through the bowel. We have conducted more than 1000 autopsies, and a lot of bodies of those who have passed away have a white, sticky coating that begins at the tongue and stretches all the way through the bowels. It's ama.

Want to see some ama? Go to a mirror, stick out your tongue, and look at it. If your tongue is coated with a white, sticky substance, that's ama.

Incomplete digestion creates ama, but it isn't the only thing that causes it. So does bad "cell digestion" (metabolism). All impurities in the functioning of the cell are ama (and wouldn't it be nice not to have them)? Ama can come from inside the body, for instance when free radicals cause damage. And it can come from outside the body, as in, for instance, "pollution." Think of anything bad in the body, and it's ama. In the blood vessels, lipids cause plaque that blocks blood flow. Another name for the accumulated lipids and plaque? Ama.

In cells, free radicals and toxins (ama) damage the cell membranes. Cells whose membranes aren't working right have trouble exchanging substances (like nutrients) with the environment around them. Cells have receptors on them that help them work with hormones and other neat chemicals in the blood stream. Damage the receptors, and those neat chemicals don't do their work.

If you damage mitochondria (small areas within the cell, usually shaped like rods), cells don't produce energy properly. Feeling a bit dragged down some days? The mitochondria probably have something to do with it. Damage the DNA (which ama can do) and you can cause mutations. You can give cancer a start.

Great, so ama is bad. Suppose you accept that. What can you do about it? Here is the connection with agni—all the different flavors of agni we mentioned. You get ama anywhere that digestion or metabolism breaks down. If you don't keep that flame working strong—in the stomach, in the liver, in the cells, between the cells, so many places—you get these toxins that Vedic medicine calls ama. Or, to put this in a positive light after all, if you do get your agni working right you won't get those toxins. It's a goal worth having.

Ama is the forerunner of all disease. If you have enough of it, you will get sick. The less of it you have, the healthier you are.

You can look at your own level of ama as an indicator (an "ama meter") of just how sick or healthy you are. Here's a brief questionnaire you can use to gauge your own level of ama:

Questionnaire: Do I Have Ama?

Circle your response (1 = least; 5 = most).

1. I tend to feel blocked in my body (constipated, congested in the head, general lack of clarity, or other).

1   2   3   4   5

2. In the morning when I wake up, I'm groggy; it takes me quite a while to feel really awake.

1   2   3   4   5

3. I tend to feel weak, physically, for no reason that I can see.

1   2   3   4   5

4. I get colds (or similar conditions) several times each year.

1   2   3   4   5

5. My body tends to have a feeling of heaviness.

1   2   3   4   5

6. I just tend to feel that "something isn't working right" in the body (digestion, breathing, bowel movements, or something else).

1   2   3   4   5

7. I tend to feel lazy. (My capacity to work seems all right, but I have no inclination.)

1   2   3   4   5

8. I commonly have indigestion.

1   2   3   4   5

9. I often have to spit.

1   2   3   4   5

10. Often, I just don't have a taste for food. I have no appetite.

1   2   3   4   5

11. I just tend to feel tired, even exhausted…in mind or body.

1   2   3   4   5

Add up your scores to arrive at a rating for your level of ama:

45 – 55	Severe
35 – 45	Moderate
25 – 35	Mild
11 – 25	Minimal

Ojas

Ama can be a depressing topic, and few lead such healthy lives that they are free of it. However, Vedic medicine also tells us of another substance, the polar opposite of ama—ojas.

Metabolism produces something. We're accustomed to thinking that the body's metabolism produces nutrients. Here's a secret from the annals of Vedic medicine. A well-functioning body, inspired by its balanced agni, produces a substance called ojas and bathes the body's cells in it.

Ojas enjoys quite an exalted position in the Vedic tradition. It's amazing stuff. It would be great if you could just glug it out of a bottle now and then, but it's so refined and pure that nobody is likely to be bottling it in the near future. Maybe the name sounds new and a little funny in the West. It sounds like "orange juice" or something that couldn't possibly be important, not like "blood." However, it's as important as you can get.

Here is some introductory information on ojas:

- Ojas, according to the ancient texts, is the essence of the tissues of your body. It pervades all over the body and regulates how everything else works. It's oily, clear, and slightly reddish yellow in color. If you lose it, you lose your body. That's it. If you keep it, your body is sure to survive. These are high stakes. Everything that can enhance ojas enriches your overall health (and overall resistance to disease, even that meanest of diseases—cancer).

- It's the master coordinator between consciousness and your body. Western medicine doesn't go beyond the physical body. For instance, it sees cancer as a disease of the physical body. Vedic medicine does venture into the "pure abstract." It sees cancer as a disease not just of the DNA, but of the consciousness that structures the DNA. Ojas coordinates the body with the body's underlying consciousness; it is the most powerful substance there is for averting cancer.

- You produce it when you have perfect digestion (which you won't get just from your single stewed apple, but it's a start).

- Metabolic processes in the physiology produce ojas. Ojas, in turn, governs metabolic processes at the junction point where the finest levels of the tissues emerge. It helps cells transform properly into healthy cells. Let's put this another way. If you don't have enough ojas, you develop a profile that sounds more or less like the citizen of the modern world. You worry a lot. (Does the term "anxiety" strike a modern cord?) You feel discomfort in the eyes, ears, and other sense organs. Your complexion gets bad (acne for some, dryness and other skin problems for any age). Your thinking goes out of whack. You may think of ojas as a funny name, but get it on your side and life goes a whole lot easier.

- Ojas nourishes your tissues beginning at their finest level.
- Ojas builds immunity. It makes your immune system (all those lymphocytes and leukocytes) balanced and stable. (You can think of the process as keeping the troops happy with good rations, plenty of recreation time, and excellent living conditions.)
- Ojas makes you strong and happy. If you increase ojas and avoid reducing it, you restore health and prevent illness. Isn't preventing illness what it's all about?

Ojas is good. Ama isn't; it causes deranged ojas, and deranged ojas causes cancer. When ojas is deranged, transformation of cells gets disturbed. You produce unwanted cells, and that is cancer.

What are some of the things that produce ama and, in the process, damage ojas? All the advice in this book, though we don't often say it that way, is to increase ojas and decrease ama. Some of the traditional advice states that you decrease the life-giving substance by anger (good old "road rage" kind of anger—that modern pastime), hunger (not such a big problem in the West, but badly timed meals and periods of hunger are common), worry, grief, and overexertion. A rough or very light diet can decrease ojas. Toxins—those noted carcinogens—tend to snuff out ojas.

Overexposure to wind and sun can deplete your precious ojas supply. Staying awake most of the night…that student favorite…deals your ojas supply a severe blow. Alcohol decimates your ojas supply. And, as many suspect but nobody wants to hear—overindulgence in sexual activity causes a major drop in that life giving, reddish yellow colored master coordinator.

If we're going to talk so much about what depletes ojas, can we flip to the other side of the coin and talk about what enriches it. Here are some suggestions:

- Anything that raises your level of consciousness. Meditation. Refined activity with the arts. Good activity with the family. Watching football on TV (well, maybe not always).
- Happiness. You should just be happy. Easier said than done, but the fact remains.—The happier you are, the more life-giving ojas you have.
- Good digestion (to which the stewed apple contributes mightily by getting the digestion off to a great start). Ojas is what you get if your digestion starts out strong and goes that way all the way through.
- Foods like milk, ghee (clarified butter), and rice in proper and limited quantity.
- Being nice (as we discuss in a complete chapter later in the book). Whole cities, some whole cultures, seem to take rudeness and coldness as right behavior. Well, those places don't culture as much ojas in their citizens as the nice places.

Begin to contemplate the power of agni, ama, and ojas, and you begin to take on a whole new attitude toward life. A gentle adjustment here and there can fill your body channels with a reddish yellow, mostly translucent fluid that is bursting with health and life and happiness.

A stewed apple in the morning gets your agni working well, which eliminates ama and enhances ojas. When you begin to think about what these benefits mean to the body, you begin to see more and more value in that humble apple. No, quercetin and boron alone are not enough to make your apple a potent cancer fighter. Get your body working right, and it can do the job. Get rid of ama, and heighten ojas, and you deliver a major blow to any cancerous tendencies anywhere in your body.

31

Three

Favor the Fighting Phytochemicals

"Yuk." Can't you just hear the word resonating in dining rooms across America as mothers place in front of their families plates of cabbage, Brussels sprouts, onions, garlic, and that longtime favorite—tofu? Traditionally no more than tolerated in the American diet (and often left on the plate even when dished out), veggies "got the power" when it comes to fighting cancer.

Although the public doesn't seem to have admitted this power to itself, science has been romancing vegetables for several years. Veggies are the darling of the scientific world. (Western medicine is fairly clueless about *how* to eat vegetables, but there Ayurveda can save the day.) Despite Western medicine's endorsement of vegetables (for all kinds of healthy purposes, including cancer prevention), society seems to be little if at all aware of what veggies can do for them. For whatever reason, people don't begin to know the amazing health power of vegetables. They are a potent cancer preventative.

Veggies: Known, Respected, Ignored

Eating vegetables has two clear benefits. First, the vegetables are healthy in themselves. The greens are rife with phytochemicals, and phytochemicals seem to be falling all over each other to benefit the body. Second, they're a "meat blocker." That is, the more you eat vegetables, the less you eat meat. Veggies are better for you than meat, but you'd hardly know it around the nation and the world. Veggies are the quiet gladiator.

Studies of vegetarians have shown again and again that you are healthier and live longer if you favor vegetables. You can find innumerable references like these words, from the Web site of physician W. Douglas Brodie, MD.—"It is a well known fact that vegetarians have a significantly lower susceptibility to cancer."

Researchers have been fond of looking at the Seventh Day Adventists, who are vegetarian. (They also don't drink alcohol, smoke, or drink coffee, which makes it a bit harder to determine just which cause is making them live longer.) They live a long time or, as one news report put it, " Seventh-Day Adventists have significantly longer-than-average life expectancies."

Where vegetables are beneficial, meat may not be such a strong cancer fighter. "New research indicates that eating lots of red meat may create about as much of a certain cancer-promoting chemical in the colon as smoking does," said one recent news report, and such an amount of the cancer-promoting chemical would be considerably too much.

One 1988 study came out bluntly under the title "Animal product consumption and mortality because of all causes combined, coronary heart disease, stroke, diabetes and cancer in Seventh-Day Adventists." The article appeared in the *American Journal of Clinical Nutrition* and found that vegetarians have the edge over meat eaters in all the mentioned disease categories.

Non-vegetarian diet can be cancer promoting in a number of ways. First of all, cooking meat forms toxins that can turn into carcinogens as they pass through your body. Also, meat eating changes the microflora (bacteria) in your intestines, which changes the process of digestion and can also lead to carcinogens. Meats can unleash hordes of free radicals in your body, too. Broiling or frying red meat turns loose oxidized compounds with the name heterocyclic amines. These guys are known mutagens. Research has found that frequent eaters of well-done meats get breast cancer more often than people who don't eat them.

Eating meat means eating less vegetables, which means you miss out on a couple of anti-cancer effects. You eat less fiber, and fiber binds carcinogens (that is, it blends with them chemically and makes them harmless). Because you eat less vegetables, you get fewer of the antioxidants in them, and by eating meat you get more heme iron (the iron found only in meat), both of which increase free radicals in the body. Besides, meat has animal fat, which can make you more obese yourself. Animal fat can change the working of your hormones for the worse (such as estrogen, often fingered as a risk in cancer). And the animal fat can suppress your immune system, which makes you less well-protected from cancer.

We're not here to alienate the many meat eaters in our audience, nor to tweak the notoriously sensitive meat lobby (who once had the temerity to challenge the American icon Oprah Winfrey herself). But we do want to point out that the word on the street (and in medical literature) is quite clear.— Vegetables are better for you than meat. It's true. It's just that nobody seems to care.

Why Veggies Are Such Good Crime Fighters

If veggies are so good, what makes them so? Phytochemicals. These plant chemicals have no nutritional value, but they do a lot of support work around the body at the chemical level. And vegetables are rife with them. (Science has discovered hundreds, and it's just getting started. As scientists continue to find and test them, phytochemicals should be attracting grants from the National Institutes of Health for years to come.)

When you look at your familiar old vegetables in the light of the potent phytochemicals in them, those old standbys take on a whole new glamour.

Phytochemicals do stuff like this:

- Prevent nasty free radicals from starting cancer
- Reduce carcinogens from being formed, such as nitrosamine (which got a lot of publicity in the 70's because bacon treated with nitrites formed nitrosamine, and meat producers had to back off on the nitrites)
- Prevent actual carcinogens that do get formed from doing their usual damage through oxidation
- Slow actual tumors from growing by slowing protein kinase C (an enzyme sometimes implicated in the growth of cancer cells)
- Protect DNA from free radical damage, inactivate carcinogens, inhibit expression of mutant genes, and activate enzyme systems involved in detoxification of toxic chemicals
- Block the cyclooxygenase enzyme, which then prevents cancer supporters named procarcinogens from actually creating cancers

This is no doubt more than you wanted to know about how vegetables do their work. The point is, a beet ain't just a beet. It's a pharmacopia. Radishes, carrots, beets, and asparagus all have chemicals in them. Eat your veggies, and you eat chemicals—good chemicals, natural chemicals, chemicals that your body likes but that damaging tendencies in the body don't like one bit. Take a look at some of the power of these natural cancer fighters.

The Broccoli Brothers

The cabbage family, sometimes called the cruciferous vegetables, is probably the most famous of the vegetable cancer fighters. Family members include cabbage, broccoli, cauliflower, mustard greens, kale, Brussels sprouts, and the increasingly popular Chinese native bok choy.

What gives these tangy veggies their punch? Indoles. Indoles block the ability of toxins to damage DNA. Indoles block the effectiveness of estrogen, quite helpful in protecting against breast cancer and uterine cancer. (The indoles are smart, too. They don't block all estrogen. They block a bad compound made from estrogen, namely 16-alpha-hydroxyestrone.) Indoles accomplish much of their good by scavenging free radicals in various ways.

Another cancer-fighter in broccoli is sulforaphane, which seems to trigger the body's own system of chemical protections against free radicals.

Also participating in the cabbage family's war of cancer prevention are isothiocyanates, which fight carcinogens and, should the need arise, cancer itself.

The cruciferous veggies have plenty of strong antioxidants, like beta-carotene, and they have flavonoids to help in the health war as well. Factor in that these veggies are high in Vitamin C as well as rich in fiber, and you have what you could definitively refer to as "a very healthy food item." For good measure, they contain Vitamin E and selenium, also antioxidants.

Fearless Leafies

It's a well-known fact that the worse things taste, the better they are for you, right? Therefore, green leafies must be really good for you. You know who they are—Swiss chard, chicory, collard greens, arugula, dandelion greens, kale, mustard greens, and spinach. Actually, it's best to make them taste delicious. But that's beside the point. As research clearly shows, these veggies' hard-earned reputation is well deserved. They're as tough on would-be cancer cells as they are unpopular at the table.

They're bursting with Vitamin C. They're rich in beta-carotene, which converts to Vitamin A. They have other carotenoids—healthful plant pigments that you can't see in the green veggies because the chlorophyll gives everything a green color. One of these carotenoids is the antioxidant lutein. A single serving has more than 100 (count 'em) different phytochemicals. What's their most famous plant pharmaceutical so far? A phytochemical whose name literally means "leaf," and that would be folate.

Folate, a B vitamin, gets right down "in the trenches" where cancer happens, because the body needs it to make DNA and RNA. It also keeps DNA healthy, resisting changes that might lead to cancer. (There is some evidence that, without folate, damage to DNA may result, which can lead to cancer.)

Drug-Wielding Tomatoes and Carrots

Hardly wanting to be left on the sidelines in the war to prevent cancer, tomatoes step forward with their own formidable weaponry. Lycopene is the new darling of gourmets, who also wouldn't mind preventing cancer. Found in tomatoes, and most effective when the tomatoes are cooked, lycopene is a front line antioxidant. It immobilizes free radicals left and right.

A physician at Harvard actually recommends that people consume tomatoes, tomato sauce, or pizza more than twice a week. His study found that such an easy-to-take regimen cut the risk of prostate cancer from between 21 to 34 percent. Other studies have found lycopene strengthening the body against cancer of the mouth, pharynx, esophagus, stomach, colon, rectum, and cervix.

Lycopene isn't the only cancer preventer in the tomato's arsenal. Tomatoes, like the leafies, have the antioxidant lutein. Until lycopene seized center stage, tomatoes were earning high praise for their beta-carotene, another potent free radical devourer.

Carrots, too, have beta-carotene, but they aren't enjoying the surge in popularity that the tomatoes and leafy greens are. Their carotenoids form Vitamin A, which, among other things, helps maintain your digestive and urinary tracts and has been linked to cancer prevention. Carrots also have vitamins B, C, D, E, and K; the minerals calcium, phosphorous, potassium, sodium, and traces of other minerals; and a trace amount of protein. That's pretty good. And they reportedly cleanse the liver.

Taking even more of a back seat than beta-carotene is the alpha-carotene found in carrots, which nevertheless is a demonstrated cancer preventer.

Gargantuan Garlic (and Unstoppable Onions)

OK, who's responsible for the surge in garlic popularity? In some circles, a gas mask is becoming a basic requirement for going to a party, because the sweet aroma of garlic hangs heavy in the air. People seem to have garlic oozing out of their pores. "If we're going to eat vegetables to fight cancer," people seem to be reasoning, "we're going to eat something that we know is having an effect on our bodies."

Well, the perception is to some degree accurate. Garlic, onions, leeks, and chives do fight cancer. Allicin is the key health builder in the garlic family. Sulfur compounds in the foods, particularly allyl sulfide, seem to block the effectiveness of cancer-causing compounds. Onions have quercetin, too, which, as we've mentioned when discussing apples, seems to nicely slow estrogen assimilation.

"A garlic a day." Have things come to this?

To further compound the frenzy around garlic, the substance seems to lower bad cholesterol as well.

Fearsome Fruits

Fruits are fighters, too. Citrus fruits have terpenes, which stimulate enzymes that block carcinogens. They have limonene, which likewise blocks carcinogens. In fact, citrus fruits contain just about every class of chemicals known for being anti-mutagenic or anti-carcinogenic.

Fruits in general have caffeic acid, which helps produce an enzyme that aids the body in discarding carcinogens. And they have ferulic acid. This brave fighter sacrifices itself by binding with nitrates, thereby (scientists theorize) preventing those chemicals from turning into cancer-causing nitrosamines.

Good Old Grains

Grains are technically vegetables. Just because they aren't

green, people tend to forget about them. But they have fiber. Oats, wheat, flax, rice, and barley have lots of dietary fiber. And they have lignans, a weak form of estrogen that takes up estrogen sites in the body (preventing stronger estrogen from being there and possibly causing cancer). Also, they have phenolic acid, believed to help in resisting breast and colon cancer. Grains count.

Yeah, But How Do You Eat Them? (Ayurveda)

Laboratories are a good place to isolate plant chemicals and see what they do at the level of the body where cancer operates—the DNA and other chemical levels. But laboratories make pretty bad kitchens.

Science seems to be pretty much at a loss in explaining *how* to eat veggies, fruits, and grains in the body's great war against cancer. "Eat all the tomatoes you can," one source will suggest, wanting you to load up on lycopene. "Eat garlic for breakfast, lunch, dinner, and in-between snacks," someone else will suggest, figuring that you can never get too much allicin. Whoever does research on a particular phytochemical seems to want you to load up on that particular one. "Eat cherries all day, they have lignans."

As important as eating fruits and veggies, is eating them right. Here are a few guidelines:

Don't Overeat Them

Traditional Ayurveda teaches that you should eat to three-quarters of capacity. Digestion, as mentioned, produces ojas—the ultimate, all-purpose cancer fighter. To digest effectively, the digestion prefers not to be overloaded. Yes, tomatoes have lycopene. That doesn't mean you should gorge yourself on tomatoes until your face turns blue. You do more harm than good for yourself if you do that.

Leave Three Hours Between Meals

"Whenever you think of it, eat another tomato," the scientific approach might suggest. "Eat garlic all day," someone might say (though we haven't literally seen such a suggestion). Digestion involves breaking down some pretty gross structures into beneficial chemicals. It takes time and concentration. It's best to leave at least three hours in between meals, so the body has the time it needs to digest your food properly. If you keep pumping more and more gross substances into the body, it makes it harder for the body to produce the refined substances that are the real cancer fighters. When the body can't produce ojas, foods become ama (toxins) instead.

Vary Them

Everybody seems to have a hobbyhorse fruit or vegetable. You have your fruitarians, your soy devotees, your tomato extremists, and your "I eat nothing but lettuce" crowd. Science doesn't have all this figured out that well. There are hundreds of cancer-preventing flavonoids, and you can find them in all kinds of fruits and vegetables. Eat a variety of them, so your body gets the benefit of a wide range of these beneficial chemicals.

Eat Them at the Right Time of Day

Onions aren't so good when you first wake up or just when you are going to bed. Most foods are best at mid-day, when digestion is highest. At other times of the day, your body may not digest these foods as well. In the quest to absorb phytonutrients, listen to your body. Don't force feed it at times when it isn't interested.

Eat the Whole Plant, not the Extract

"Tomatoes have lycopene; I think I'll take lycopene tablets," people might tend to think. But any fruit or vegetable, made in nature, is a rich stew of nutrients and phytochemicals where "the whole is greater than the sum of the parts." Sometimes an isolated ingredient, such as ascorbic acid (Vitamin C), doesn't have nearly the benefit that, say, a whole orange will have. Sometimes it can even have a negative effect.

Do Cook Them

The health food movement has one faction that believes you should not cook vegetables. However, some people have difficulty digesting raw vegetables and end up with a belly full of gas. Cooking vegetables is good for the vegetables and good for you. You can much more readily digest the vegetables and turn them into phytonutrients if you help your digestion by cooking the veggies in the first place.

But Don't Charbroil Them

Why is it that "restaurant" and "healthy food" seem to be opposites. Restaurants can take almost anything and make it unhealthy. Yes, a charbroiled onion may taste better than a boiled one, but charbroiling produces potential carcinogens. Eat a charbroiled item now and then, if you wish, but favor more gentle cooking methods on the whole. If you use some spices to prepare your veggies, they will taste just as delicious and do your body good.

Veggies. They're beginning to have their day, and they are awesome cancer fighters. Their benefit is not just folk wisdom any more. Vegetables have indoles in them. They have lycopene, quercetin, and fearsome folates. They have isoflavones, alpha-carotene, and beta-carotene. At the nitty gritty chemical level where the cancer prevention war takes place, they are fearsome fighters. Eat them.

❧ Four

Try Anti-Tumor Turmeric

I s there one, magical, cure-all anti-cancer herb…one that you could just "take" if you really didn't want to read everything about anti-cancer approaches? Is there just one herb that soothes the cells, stimulates the right enzymes, and protects the intelligence of the cell's DNA? One that is delicious? Cheap? Available over the counter at the supermarket?

If so, what would it be? Would that magical protector be the widely acclaimed Chinese green tea? Would it be the ferociously named "cat's claw?" Would it be that potent, much-debated substance—garlic—that hits your system so hard you know it has to be doing something (and you hope it's good)? That clearly spicy, attention-getting ginger?

Yes, there is a top anti-cancer herb, and, no, it is none of the fad favorites just mentioned (though those also have their value). Ayurveda's top candidate as the world's best anti-cancer herb would be nothing other than the commonplace turmeric. Yes, *that* turmeric, the one that for years seemed like just a little food coloring. In the recent past, if you had it at all, it sat on the shelf in the same bottle for month after month and year

43

after year until you moved away, cleaned house, and threw it out. Little, orange, tasteless, neglected turmeric. It's a serious cancer fighter.

Neglected in the West, turmeric has been a pillar of the diet in India for thousands of years. There in the East the bottle does not sit neglected, and turmeric is hardly just food coloring. For at least 5,000 years—every day in every Indian kitchen, while cooking their lentils and vegetables with turmeric—Indians have been using this anti-cancer wonder spice.

Ayurvedic tradition knows both the herb itself and, just as important, how to use it to coax the maximum benefit from the seemingly shy herb. Need a little convincing on the possible benefits of this "sleeper"—a relative of the much more zesty ginger plant and, like ginger, derived from the root of the plant? You can get it now from Western medicine, which recently has devoted a good deal of research to the subject of this now-remembered spice. Here from Western science are some of the documented benefits of curcumin (turmeric's top enhancing ingredient, known technically as diferuloyl methane), as cited by Thomas M. Newmark and Paul Schulick:

- More DNA protective than [powerful antixoidants] lipoate, vitamin E and beta carotene
- Stimulates glutathione S-transferase, a detoxifying, cancer-protective enzyme
- Modulates nitric oxide and is associated with its anti-inflammatory and anti-cancer activities
- Strongly anti-inflammatory, both orally and topically, and, like green tea and *Ocimum sanctum,* is anti-ulcerative
- Intensifies the anti-cancer activity of other phytonutrients [plant chemicals]
- Inhibits leukemia at initiation, promotion and progression
- Inhibits precancerous colon lesions
- Inhibits the growth of multiple breast cancer cell lines
- Suppresses colon cancer

- Inhibitory of oral tumors
- Topically applied curcumin can strongly inhibit skin tumor promotion

If that list isn't enough to spark your interest, here are some more of turmeric's healthful qualities:

- Antibacterial activity in its turmeric oil
- Enhances metabolism (i.e., good for digestion)
- Protects against heart disease

Turmeric is good for your digestion, which means that it will help to dissolve those undesirable fats in your body instead of allowing them to accumulate. It gobbles up free radicals, which protects your blood vessels. It's antibacterial, and it's always good for the heart to cut down on the infection-causing bacteria in the system. And it is a supremo antioxidant. Would you have thought that it's good for your heart, to eat turmeric regularly as a cancer-preventative? Well, it is.

"Wow," you might think, "this flat-tasting, slightly bitter, yellow-orange powder can do all that? Who would have guessed it? I'll take a spoonful with every meal." The stuff is cheap and available. You might be tempted to load it into a water bottle and glug it all day long. And, as a natural food, it seems perfectly harmless. Why not just eat as much as you want? Well, these initial reactions deserve a bit more attention, along with one other common perception of such a potent herb.—"If this stuff does all this, why don't I just extract the potent part, and have a genuine drug for myself?" First, let's start with the right way to use turmeric. Then we'll lay to rest some of the popular misconceptions surrounding it.

Cook with It

First of all, there are right ways and wrong ways to ingest your turmeric. The right way (you won't find this advice hard to swallow) is to cook with it. According to the ancient Ayurvedic tradition, the best way to use this potent spice is also the way that it tastes best and is easiest to digest. Eating deliciously cooked turmeric doesn't just get your own gastric juices flowing (which helps you assimilate the herb and get the most benefit from it). The cooking itself also brings out the best in the substance. When you cook turmeric with food, the turmeric doesn't lose any of its innate, plant intelligence. Instead, the intelligence of the turmeric enhances the intelligence of the food, and vice versa. Food and turmeric play a very pleasant duet together, to the lasting benefit of your body.

Turmeric goes with every kind of taste identified by Ayurveda. This substance is versatile. You can put it in a salty dish, which you may not find surprising, but you can also put it in a sweet dish.

Create a Turmeric Sauce for Everyday Use

To create a versatile sauce with turmeric, sauté the turmeric in olive oil or ghee (clarified butter), then put it on your food. You can add turmeric to any of your foods. The serving size is ¼ tsp. per meal.

Note that some of turmeric's beneficial nutrients are water-soluble and some are fat-soluble. By sautéing with ghee or olive oil, you release the fat-soluble chemicals. By mixing with food and cooking, you release the water-soluble chemicals. It's best to do both.

Cook it with Your Main Meal

Cook lentils, vegetables, fish, poultry, and other meats with turmeric. Most popular curries from India include turmeric, and curries are indeed a great way to get your medicinal benefits while indulging in a delectable meal. Here's a tasty curry recipe:

Curry

Ingredients:
   6 parts turmeric
   10 parts ground cumin
   1 part ground *ajwan*

6 parts ground fennel

1 part ground black pepper

(Ajwan, if it's new to you, is an excellent anti-cancer spice, good for cleaning out the channels in the body. You can get it at an Indian grocery.)

Directions:

1. Mix the spices together well.
2. Use this mixture when cooking your lentils, vegetables, or meats. A recommended serving size is ½ to 1 tsp. per person. Enjoy this curry with lunch and dinner.
3. Store the spice mixture in an airtight container in a cool place away from direct sunlight.

Here's a good way to cook vegetables with this spice mixture:

1. Heat up a little oil or ghee on medium to medium-high heat.
2. Add the spice mixture and sauté briefly.
3. Add the vegetables and stir them into the spice mixture.
4. Add water if necessary, add salt, and continue cooking until done.

This method maximizes the healthful effects of the spices and also makes the veggies taste so good you'll actually want to eat them!

Enjoy Delicious Turmeric Milk

Here's a way to enjoy turmeric in liquid form. Besides preventing cancer, this tasty delight helps prevent colds.

Add ¼ tsp. turmeric to one cup of milk and boil it. Then sip it slowly.

Make Your Own Immunity Booster

You can mix together several spices, including turmeric, to strengthen your immunity to colds, flu, and all kinds of other imbalances. Here's how to make your own Immunity Mix:

Immunity Mix

Ingredients:

6 parts turmeric
3 parts ground cumin
3 parts ground coriander
6 parts ground fennel
1 part powdered dry ginger
1 part ground black pepper
¼ part ground cinnamon

Directions:

1. Mix the spices together well. (Store them in an airtight container in a cool place away from direct sunlight.)
2. Heat one teaspoon of the spice mixture in one tablespoon of ghee, using medium to medium-high heat, until the mixture releases an aroma. Remove from the heat immediately, so it won't burn.
3. Put this spiced ghee on cooked rice, vegetables, or your other foods. (Or you can cook your vegetables with this spice mixture the same way as mentioned above.)

If you take this combination of spices regularly with each main meal of the day, you'll boost your immune system and enhance your digestion.

Don't Miss Turmeric When on the Road

Travel a lot? You don't have to be deprived of turmeric just because you're eating in airports and ordering from room service at a hotel. Here's how to make turmeric you can take with you:

Turmeric to Go

Directions:

1. Bring one tablespoon of ghee to a boil.
2. When the ghee starts to boil, put in one teaspoon turmeric powder. Start stirring immediately.
3. When the mixture starts turning brown, remove it from the heat and continue stirring.

4. Keep stirring until it cools down.

5. Store in a glass bottle. It will stay fresh, unrefrigerated, for at least one week.

6. Sprinkle it on your food when you're on the road. Use ¼ tsp. per meal.

Don't Overdo it

Turmeric is hardly one of those pharmaceuticals you can easily overdose on. It's food, not a prescription drug. But tradition does talk about the right amount to take—about a quarter teaspoonful per meal, cooked with your food.

When should you not take it at all? Turmeric stimulates the liver, making it more effective in producing bile. If you have any kind of a blockage in the bile duct, "cool it" with the turmeric (that is, don't take turmeric). The herb could aggravate the situation, with the liver making more bile and the duct unable to allow it to pass through.

If you don't have a blocked bile duct, can you eat as much turmeric as you want? Again, moderation is best. In India, where people have been eating turmeric over the centuries, they're used to it. But too much turmeric (i.e. more than the small dosages we've just recommended) can create too much "heat" for the liver. Turmeric may not seem hot to you. As mentioned, it tastes bitter but hardly hot like a chili or something. As Ayurveda explains, turmeric is actually hot in its effect, because it stimulates digestion and wakes up the liver. Overdo it, and you can create an imbalance, experiencing such effects as hunger, a short temper, or irritability.

"Hey, Why Not Just Extract the Good Stuff?"

Like many other popular herbs, turmeric has attracted the attention of the marketers. Some companies extract just the curcumin, and you can take it in pill form. According to Ayurveda, the cold, hard, medicinal approach isn't as good as the gentle approach. Ayurveda recommends having your turmeric as the complete herb and not as an extract.

First of all, the full-strength, extracted herb can overburden the physiology just as too much straight turmeric might do. Second, turmeric is more than just the curcumin that the scientists identify as its enhancing ingredient. Stripping away its accompanying ingredients is like cutting Samson's hair. The herb loses power. As Newmark and Schulick point out, "a highly isolated turmeric extract standardized only to curcumin would miss the recognized cancer-preventative and anti-inflammatory properties present in the whole plant."

Western medicine confirms the longstanding practice of Ayurveda to work with whole plants. Whereas whole turmeric is antioxidant, isolated curcumin can actually allow oxidants (free radicals) to have increased damaging effects. Here's another piece of information that gives us pause. Turmeric stimulates glutathione S-transferase (GST), an enzyme that carries out detoxification. But isolated curcumin, in high doses, can actually suppress GST. It's a rather chilling thought, but the extract can have the opposite effect of the whole herb.

Ayurveda in general prefers whole plants to extracts. Ayurveda looks to culture "wholeness"—the full expression of what nature has provided. Whether you are eating spices, grains, vegetables, or fruits, Ayurveda recommends eating them whole and fresh. The body itself is whole, not fragmented. Fresh, whole foods provide holistic support to the body for holistic results.

Often the chemical extraction method kills the intelligence of the plant. If the method itself doesn't have that effect, then the isolation will do it. Cancer prevention has everything to do with preserving and strengthening cell intelligence, preventing cells from losing contact with their own intelligence and going berserk. Therefore, processes that damage cell intelligence defeat the intended purpose.

Turmeric. Would you ever have made it your first choice as a potent anti-cancer substance? It is completely unassuming.

The beauty of this quiet champion is that it does its good work without you noticing anything except perhaps the delicious taste of foods cooked with it.

Ironically, all the ways you are supposed to take it are the ways that most people in their normal state of mind would like to take it. Cook it so that it tastes good. Don't go looking for ways to eat a lot of it. (You'll just annoy your liver.) Don't bother with the expensive extracts you can order on the Internet. Cook with it every day, and enjoy its benefits for easing digestion, fighting those damaging free radicals, improving blood flow, and literally preventing tumors before they start.

Turmeric. Boy, that's some food coloring.

PART TWO

&

Key "Don't Die Yet" Methods

Five

The "Don't Die Yet" Diet

OK, it's time to lay to rest a notion—namely that healthy meals taste bad. Sure, all those prepackaged diet meals taste bad, but they aren't really that healthy. Raw mustard greens aren't going to float anybody's boat either. Celery shake? Yuk.

In fact, the healthiest meals you can make also taste the best. If they don't taste really great, they aren't healthy. Really. Here's how that works. You see, if something tastes great, you salivate over it prodigiously. Your other gastric juices get pumping away spontaneously.—Stomach acid. Just the right amount of bile. Everything gets working. Then you digest better, produce more nutrients, and make fewer toxins.

You should be happy while you're eating. That's not just a moral stricture. If you're happy, you have positive neuropeptides floating around in your body. Positive neuropeptides help you digest better. Again, you create more positive chemicals in your body and fewer toxins. Happiness is a digestive aid.

On the other hand, food that tastes yucky is bad for digestion and, if you repeat it often enough, could even be a carcinogen.

Stuff that "turns your stomach" just doesn't get digested well, and that wreaks havoc throughout your system. For starters, it sits in the colon and tries to attach bad stuff to the linings there. It sends free radicals catapulting through the system looking for healthy molecules to attack. It's not good. It makes you sick in the long run, and sometimes in the short run, too.

So, if you were beginning to steel yourself to a bad tasting meal as you began this chapter, forget about it. The word "anti-cancer," we'll admit, is an unappetizing word and gets us off to a bad start. We'd rather use some nice word, such as "pro-health," but we don't want anyone to miss the point. We are talking here about a meal that prevents cancer. It's just that you don't have to be thinking at all about preventing cancer as you eat it. (In fact, since preventing cancer isn't an appetizing subject, you'd best ignore the issue as you eat.)

The Munificent Meal

It's best to have your main meal of the day at noon, when the digestive fire is highest. Here's what to put on the plate of your sumptuous meal, which is nevertheless quite easy and quick to prepare. Once we've given you the big picture, we'll break it down component by delectable component in the rest of the chapter:

- A small piece of ginger to awaken the appetite before you begin
- Some nice, whole grain, such as rice
- A nicely spiced bean dish, such as *dal* (chicken instead for the non-veggies)
- Green, leafy veggies
- Flat bread (known as *chapati* or *roti*)
- Green, leafy *chutney*
- Fresh cheese (*panir*)
- Nuts, perhaps walnuts
- Fruit and dates
- A nice, gentle sweet
- *Lassi*

That's the meal. Eat it every day for lunch, and you'll do wonders for your health. You can vary lots of the participants, so it doesn't become boring. You can have all kinds of whole grains, various veggies, numerous nuts, and so on. And, with a few spices and the right preparation, the combination is a taste delight (way, way more sumptuous than, say, a Big Mac from McDonald's).

Jolly Ginger

To make sure your digestion is wide awake and ready to roll, take a thin slice of fresh ginger root and sprinkle it with a little salt. Eat this right before you start your meal to put your digestion on high alert.

A Wholesome Whole Grain

Whole grains are healthy, but most people aren't even too sure what they are. It's hard to tell the whole ones from the partial ones. Whole grains keep their fiber, their vitamins, and their minerals like zinc and potassium, whereas processed grains lose some. The complete grains have antioxidants, lignans, phenolic acids, and other phytochemicals. They are rich in the very things we've been talking about for preventing cancer, where your partial grains come along with much of those things stripped out. If cancer-prevention is your game, whole grains should be your choice. The fiber will have its anti-cancer effect by enhancing digestion, and other phytochemicals in the whole grain will aid in your ongoing cancer prevention battle.

Here are some good whole grains to choose from:
- Barley
- Couscous
- Millet
- Quinoa
- Rye
- Rice

Prepare your rice so that it is cooked but still firm and the grains don't stick together. *Basmati rice,* available at Indian groceries and most health food stores, is the king of all rices. It's a high-quality long-grain rice that has a unique aroma when cooked. Here's one way to prepare Basmati rice:

Basmati Rice

Directions:
1. Wash the rice in several changes of cold water.
2. Put the rice in a saucepan and add 1 ½ times as much water as you have rice.
3. Bring to a boil, then stir, cover the pan, and reduce to a simmer.
4. Simmer gently for 10 minutes.
5. Remove the pan from the heat and let it sit covered for 5 minutes.
6. Fluff the rice with a fork and serve.

Beneficent Beans

Often overlooked in American cookery, to be served with franks on a picnic, beans are a potent nutritional player in the anti-cancer diet. First, they have protein. You don't have to eat meat to get protein. You help your cause a lot if you eat beans, dals, and lentils. Second, this family of foods (which we simplify to just "beans") also has fiber, like grains. So, in having beans, you're doubling up your beneficial fiber. Third, beans have complex carbohydrates and vitamins.

You can use them all kinds of ways: appetizers, salads, soups, main dishes, sides, and even dessert. You've had rice pudding before, right? Well, beans can be used in desserts as well.

If you want to choose a favorite, the Vedic medical tradition gives a nod to mung beans, the split ones with the skins removed (which are referred to as *moong dal* in Indian groceries). They're easier to digest than most of the other beans and dals. You can eat them every day without any bad consequences.

Here are some other nutritious beans, which you can get at a health food store or an Indian grocery:

- *Toor dal*—this yellow bean is quite nourishing and mixes very well with vegetables.
- *Chana dal*—yellow like the Toor dal, this one holds its shape even when it's fully cooked. Many enjoy its nutty flavor.
- *Urad dal*—This one you can get either split and hulled, or split with the skins still on.

Here's some anti-cancer advice on cooking with beans:

- Cook them. (This one keeps coming up.) When they're well cooked, the digestion can get down right away to its task of transforming them into beneficial chemicals.
- Sort through them a bit before you cook them. You'll probably find an occasional small stone to remove.
- Rinse them several times before you cook them.
- Contrary to popular practice in the West, don't add salt before the beans are cooked. Acidic ingredients like tomatoes or lemon juice shouldn't go in either until you've cooked the beans. Then add these things and cook a few more minutes.
- What you can add are spices like cumin, black pepper, and ginger (which has demonstrated anti-cancer effects).
- For some beans, you should soak them for a while first to soften them up before cooking.
- To store your dry beans and dals, keep them in dry, airtight containers at normal room temperature.
- Beans keep, but try to use them within six months or so. As they get older, they lose moisture and take longer to soak and cook.

Here's a nice, basic recipe:

Split Moong Dal

(2 servings)

Ingredients:

½ cup split moong dal

2 cups water
½ teaspoon salt
¼ carrot, cut into thin slices
½ teaspoon fresh ginger root, grated
1 teaspoon Immunity Mix (see Chapter 4)
1 tablespoon ghee (clarified butter)
1 teaspoon fresh cilantro leaves, chopped
½ teaspoon fresh lemon juice

Directions:

1. Sort through the dal and remove any small stones, then rinse the dal in cool water several times.
2. Put the water, carrots, and dal in a medium-sized saucepan, and bring it to a boil. (If foam forms on the top of the boiling water, skim it off and throw it away.)
3. Lower the heat, and continue to simmer the dal for 20 minutes until it is tender. (If you like a thicker dal, continue the boiling for another 5 minutes.)
4. Add the salt.
5. Melt the ghee in a separate saucepan. Add the ginger root, and sauté for several minutes. Add the Immunity Mix and sauté briefly, about 30 seconds, with the ginger root. (Be sure that you don't burn the spices.)
6. Add the spice mixture to the dal and stir. (Be careful. The dal may splash a little when you put in the hot oil.)
7. Add the lemon juice and fresh cilantro. Stir and serve.

Generous Greens

The dark green leafy vegetables, half-scorned in Western cookery as Popeye's strength builder, hold a high position as a cancer fighter. As we've explained in Chapter 3, they have beta-carotene, other carotenoids, lutein (an unyielding antioxidant), and—above all—DNA-enriching folate. They're rich in minerals like calcium and Vitamin A.

Vedic medicine has known about them forever and has held them in high esteem. Know what they have that Western medicine is just beginning to measure? *Prana* (another one of those Vedic terms), which is pure life energy. Prana is the antithesis of cancer. Also, according to the Vedic approaches, they have juices in them that keep your body nice and fluid.— They keep open subtle channels in the body where nutrients have to flow if they're going to keep cells strong.

Here are some green leafies you'll enjoy:

- Bok choy
- Collard greens
- Kale
- Mustard greens
- Sorrel
- Spinach
- Swiss chard
- Turnip greens

Different greens have different cooking requirements, of course. Some (spinach) are pretty tender and cook fast. Others (kale) take longer to get tender. But do cook them. Otherwise, your stomach may complain.

Here are two simple recipes that get your cancer fighting forces working:

Prana Dal

(Recipe for 3)

Ingredients:

    1 cup moong dal
    1 lb. fresh organic spinach
    ½ teaspoon turmeric
    Pinch of ground coriander
    Pinch of ground cumin
    Pinch of ground ginger
    Salt to taste
    ½ teaspoon fresh lemon juice
    A few pinches of black salt (actually looks pink, available at an Indian grocery store)

61

Directions:

1. Sort through the dal and remove any small stones, then rinse the dal in cool water several times.
2. Cook the dal with the turmeric, coriander, cumin, and ginger. You should have approx. 2 ½ cups of thin cooked dal when done.
3. Add salt to taste and cook a few more minutes.
4. Wash the spinach thoroughly, then lightly steam it for 2-3 minutes.
5. Put the dal and spinach in a blender, and blend for only 2-3 seconds, just enough to distribute the spinach throughout the dal without turning it into liquid.
6. Pour into serving bowls. Sprinkle with fresh lemon juice and a pinch of black salt. Serve it with rice or a chapati.

Sautéed Swiss Chard

Ingredients:

1 lb. Swiss chard, finely chopped
1 tablespoon ghee
1 teaspoon Immunity Mix (see Chapter 4)
Salt to taste
½ teaspoon lemon juice

Directions:

1. Heat the ghee in a frying pan.
2. Sauté the Immunity Mix in the ghee very briefly, about 40 seconds, on low heat.
3. Add the Swiss chard and stir it into the spices.
4. Add about 2 tablespoons of water and cover the pan. Cook for about 10 minutes, until the Swiss chard is tender.
5. Add salt and lemon juice. Cook for a few more minutes, then serve.

Bountiful Bread

Know what's good about chapatis (flat breads)? You can use them instead of silverware. In some places in the West, people frown on such behavior. It's standard in the East, where touching the food is considered an integral part of the dining experience. Chapatis also taste good and contribute to the delight of the meal. You can buy them in the store or, if you have time, make them yourself.

Satisfying Sides

Enjoyment is an essential part of a delightful anti-cancer meal. Remember, you're trying to keep the celebration of life going on in your body at even its most quiet levels (well, all right, especially at its most quiet levels). To do that, you should keep pleasing your tastes in all kinds of ways. Variety is good. And spice is the variety of life. For instance, a nicely spiced chutney is almost a requirement for your anti-cancer meal.

Chutney

There are a wide variety of chutneys to accompany your meals. Some are made with spices and cooked fruits. Others are made using cilantro, mint, or coconut. They do all kinds of good things for digestion, besides making the meal a lot more fun for your taste buds and for the rest of you. You can purchase them rather than making them yourself, and have a little with your meal.

Fresh Cheeses Such as Panir or Ricotta

Panir, if you aren't familiar with it yet, is great. It's very popular with those who do know it, because it's light and easy to digest, yet bursting with the nutritional value of cheese. (Some cheeses you buy at the grocery store may be aged and can produce free radicals in the body, which are harmful to the physiology. They are also very heavy and can clog up your system.) You might find panir at an Indian grocery, or you can make it yourself. Here's the recipe:

Panir

Ingredients:

1 quart of milk (not homogenized is better)
Juice of 1 squeezed lemon

Directions:

1. Bring the milk to a boil.
2. Add the lemon juice. (The milk will start to curdle, but in this case that's what you want.)
3. Turn off the heat and let the substance sit for a few moments, then bring it back to boiling.
4. Remove it from the heat. When it is half-cool, strain the curds from the whey through any fine cloth. (Muslin is good, or several layers of cheesecloth.)
5. When most of the moisture has drained, gather the top of the cloth, tie it together, and hang it somewhere to drip. Let all the water drip through (which usually takes about an hour).

Yield: One cup of panir. You can cook it in with your veggies for a delicious and nutritious dish.

If you are going to make fresh cheese yourself, we recommend the panir. A similar cheese you can also make is ricotta; you can find recipes for it on the Internet. Ricotta is often available in grocery stores; if not, fresh cottage cheese will do.

Nuts

Don't forget to toss in a few nuts with your meal. Nuts keep falling in and out of favor with the diet crowd. "Oh, they have protein. That's good. Oh, they have too much fat. That's bad." In our crowd, they're good. Besides adding protein, know what they can do? Feed your brain, and the brain is the main switchboard for everything going on in your body. Walnuts have the healthy Omega-3 fats. It's best to soak your walnuts overnight before eating them, which removes a certain sharpness from them that makes them harder to digest.

Other nutritious nuts are sesame seeds (toasted), sunflower seeds, and almonds (blanched).

Here's a delicious, nutty recipe you can eat with your evening meal:

Nutty Delight

Ingredients:
  2 parts sesame seeds, hulled
  1 part white poppy seeds
  1 part dried coconut (fresh, if you can get it)

Directions:
1. Soak everything together for about an hour, until it's soft.
2. Blend the mixture into a smooth paste.
3. Add this nutty paste to your vegetables or other foods as you cook them. Allow a tablespoon of paste per serving.

This mixture will help you sleep, and you'll wake up ready to attack the day with vigor.

Death-Defying Desserts

The anti-cancer devotee can be understandably reluctant about desserts. Don't desserts have processed sugars, which can be carcinogens (as we explain in a later chapter of this book)? Don't they have fats? Aren't they downright sinful? Not always, and it's important to indulge your tastes, as we said. A dissatisfied body is a body wont to fall sick. Have some tasty, fresh desserts. Here are some suggestions:

Fruit

Fresh or cooked fruits are great for after the meal. Have pears, apples, oranges, peaches, cherries, blueberries, mangoes, bananas. Whatever is in season is best. Dried fruits are great, too—apricots, dates, figs, raisins. An ideal after-dinner fruit is an organic *Medjool* date. (If you've never had an organic Medjool date, you've never really had a date.) Their sumptuous richness can change your mind forever in favor of that fruit. You won't be able to eat just one. Two to four should meet your needs nicely.

Some Sumptuous Sweet

Some other delicious sweet following the meal is good. Rice pudding is an excellent choice. Especially if it's made with organic milk and raw sugar (instead of processed white sugar).

Lassi

For your noon meal, lassi can be a great aid to digestion. (It's better not to have it in the evening, though.) Drink the lassi after you finish eating. Lassi is made by mixing fresh yogurt with water, and adding a few other tasty ingredients. Yogurt in its native form tends to clog digestion a bit. But when you blend it with water and make it into lassi, it aids digestion. The reason for this is that blending thins the yogurt and changes its molecular structure.

There are many recipes for lassi. Here are three for you to choose from:

Sweet Lassi

Ingredients:
   1 part cold yogurt
   3 parts water
   Pinch of ground cardamom
   Pinch of sugar
   Splash of rosewater

Directions:

Blend all ingredients together. Include cardamom, sugar, and rosewater, to taste. Drink after lunch.

Digestive Lassi

Ingredients:
   1 part cold yogurt
   3 parts water
   Pinch of ground ginger
   Pinch of ground cumin
   Pinch of salt
   Pinch of black pepper

Directions:

Blend all ingredients together. Include ginger, cumin, salt, and pepper, to taste. Drink after lunch.

Lassi to prevent gas, bloating

Ingredients:

1 cup room-temperature water
¼ cup fresh homemade yogurt
1 pinch ground ginger
1 pinch ground cumin
1 pinch ground coriander
1 pinch salt

Directions:

Blend everything together for one minute. Drink after lunch to ward off gas and bloating.

A Couple of Culinary Cautions

People don't like somebody watching them as they eat. "Keep your eyes on your own plate" is excellent folk wisdom for avoiding annoyance and other forms of consternation at the dinner table. People don't like to be told how to eat, either.

We'd nevertheless like to pass along a few tried-and-true approaches from the Vedic tradition, practices said to have been followed by the longest-living people in the past. You don't have to follow all of these suggestions all of the time. But if you review them and gently move yourself in their direction, you'll help make your digestion optimum.

Here are our humble bits of advice:

■ **Eat your main meal in the middle of the day**

Digestion is the objective. Maximum objective. In the middle of the day, agni is primed and ready. Your body, supported by the whole of nature, is most prepared to digest food. By a similar token, it's better not to eat a heavy meal in the evening. Some light soup and bread is good at that time.

Even when eating at mid-day, help your digestion by eating the hardest to digest things first—heavy desserts, fried foods, salad. The digestive fire is strongest before it has been working on other foods.

It's also good to be in the habit of eating at the same time each day. The body loves that regularity and knows when to have its juices ready for digestion, then it can focus its attention on finer levels of activity.

■ Don't eat too much

Overeating is a great Western sport. People eat until they're stuffed, then eat a little more, topped off by dessert. When you eat that much, your digestion doesn't have room to do optimum work. Some foods get only partially digested (i.e. turn into ama). It's best to eat to ¾ of your capacity.

Also, once your digestion gets working after one meal, it's best to let it run its course without asking it to keep starting over and over with additional food items. Usually wait two to three hours after one meal before eating something additional.

■ Sit down while you eat

Some of these suggestions sound so obvious that you'd think we'd be embarrassed to say them. In one chapter we found ourselves advising people to sleep at night. Now here we are saying that people should sit down while they eat. Aren't these things obvious? Well, with the passage of time, they seem to have been partially overlooked. Airports let you eat your sandwich at a stand-up counter. The symphony serves finger foods, and expects you to eat them while standing.

The general idea with our time-honored recommendation is to take a load off your feet and your mind for awhile as you eat, so that your stomach, brain, and overall digestive system can focus their energies on the task at hand—turning your food into nutrients instead of useless particles floating around in the body.

■ Don't watch TV while you eat

Yes, it's refreshing to see one more nostalgic episode of "I Dream of Jeannie," but watching TV absorbs the brain. Your brain forgets to guide you in breaking down and distributing your foods. It's better to focus all your attention on your meal. You'll enjoy your food much more, and digest it better too.

■ **Don't read while you eat**

Go into a restaurant on the road, and you hear it all the time—"I'll take coffee, two donuts, and the *USA Today.*" Well, the newspaper is just as distracting as TV. Sure, it may be embarrassing at first to sit there in public alone with your food. But you can get used to it, and your digestion will certainly appreciate it.

There are some similar cautions, such as—don't eat while driving. Aside from the inherent dangers involved, the reason for not eating while driving is that the road takes your body's attention away from the key task at hand—digesting.

■ **Don't argue with someone or do business while you eat**

Arguing or doing business is a step worse than just reading while you eat. You want your stomach producing nice things as it digests—positive neuropeptides that create bliss throughout the body. Arguments and business create various stress hormones and, in general, turn the stomach. You can't avoid emotional upsets all the time, but try to avoid them during meals.

■ **Combat the trend to ice-cold beverages and food**

The "agni fire" of digestion. Obviously, the West doesn't know about it. When you eat, you want to have your digestive fire nicely burning away so you can transform your food into nutrients. Cold puts out the fire. Ice really puts it out. Ice is the antithesis of digestion, but nobody in the mainstream of food seems to recognize that yet.

Somebody ought to advise American Airlines. When the steward walks down the aisle with his drinks, the plastic glasses are always full of ice. You have to ask him to dump the ice, and he has trouble not looking annoyed when you do. Your favorite white-table-cloth restaurant is no better. At your seat when you sit down are glasses filled with ice water. Ask for water without ice, and they'll just fish the cubes out of your ice-cold water (which really misses the point). When you sip a little (and douse your digestive fire in the process), the always-attentive waiter comes around to clink more ice water into your glass.

The only alternative to hot tea in a restaurant is "iced tea." You can't just have room-temperature tea. Buy a water bottle from your local Seven Eleven, and the store thinks it's doing you a favor by keeping it in the cooler. Ask for room-temperature water, and a salesclerk eyebrow shoots up as if you're a weirdo. People seem to think that room temperature water doesn't quench thirst, but it really does.

Ice. Ice. Ice. America thinks it is inseparable from drinks, but in reality, it chills the flavor, chills your belly, chills your liver, and slows digestion just when you need it most. Go on a campaign to avoid ice. Don't just order "lemonade," order "lemonade, no ice."

■ Avoid these foods:

- Leftovers

  While avoiding ice, also avoid another popular favorite—leftovers. Some home cooks, yes, are masters of making those eggs from breakfast be great at lunch and having the boiled potatoes from lunch one day be great as fried potatoes two days later. But the older foods lose their vitality and become harder to digest.

- Processed foods

  Skip right by the frozen pizza aisle in the supermarket. In fact, pass up most of the aisles in the middle. Processed foods tend to have a lot of chemical additives. They are also lacking in vitality. Stick with the fresh foods.

- Fast foods

  The healthy ingredients get steamrollered as the chains make their foods so fast. The prana gets suffocated. Fast foods are also generally high in salt or high in fat or both.

- Foods with additives or artificial ingredients

  You want the real nutrients—the phytonutrients and vitamins and minerals. And you don't want anything that may turn into toxins.

A delightful meal is an anti-cancer meal. And an anti-cancer meal is a delightful meal. Your greens, dals, nuts, and chutneys are so lively they are a symphony awaiting you on the plate.

Eat a potent anti-cancer meal at noon every day, and toxins won't know where to collect in your body. Meantime, positive chemicals will go coursing through you, opening up channels and delighting the brain.

Forget these "Fighting" (Contradictory) Foods

We don't like bringing this up in mixed company, but we feel that we have to…in the interest of preventing a lot of future indigestion in our readership. Look, some foods just can't get along with one another. You can't let them in the stomach at the same time. That's just the way it is. They curdle, annoy, stifle, or otherwise rile the other food. That might be all right if it were happening in a test tube somewhere, but you don't want it going on in your stomach.

Here is a partial list that has been developed, to help avoid the most common mistakes in food-combining found in the Western countries. Clearly, there are a lot more foods that don't get along than the few we have here.

Here's what to do.—Leave at least an hour between eating foods that are incompatible with each other. That's the basic guideline. You don't have to strain to do these things, just quietly have the intention. You don't have to stop altogether right away with your orange juice milkshakes. (Well, maybe you should.) But cut the orange juice in the shake a little bit each day until, voilà, there is none there.

1. Do not combine milk with:
   • Meals that have mixed tastes, e.g. vegetables
   • Sour foods, e.g. sour fruits, yogurt, etc.
   • Fermented foods of any kind, e.g. apple cider, soy sauce, etc.
   • Fermented herbal supplements, e.g. tinctures, etc.
   • Pickled foods, e.g. gherkins and many Indian condiments
   • Vinegar, or salad dressings containing vinegar
   • Citrus fruits—oranges, grapefruit, pineapple, lemons, limes, etc.

- Green leafy vegetables—spinach, kale, broccoli, arugula, etc.
- Radish
- Eggs of any kind
- Baked foods containing eggs, e.g. breads, cakes, cookies
- Meat of any kind—beef, chicken, pork, turkey, fish, etc.
- Garlic
- Salt
- Foods containing salt, e.g. most processed foods, fish, sea vegetables, crackers, peanuts, etc.
- Alcohol

We know this list sounds all-inclusive at first, as in, "Fine, then when can I drink my milk?" Most people who have been following Vedic guidelines for a while don't drink milk along with their meals. They drink milk. They have it before bedtime. They have it in the late afternoon as a picker upper. Milk is good, but you have to watch the company that it keeps.

While we're on the subject, milk is much easier to digest if you boil it first. Organic milk is recommended. The cows that produce this milk were not given bovine growth hormone, and the food they ate didn't contain pesticides, herbicides, or antibiotics. You should also use pasteurized milk that is not homogenized. Homogenized milk clogs the fine channels of the body, the very ones your anti-cancer approaches seek to free up.

2. Use raw (uncooked) honey only. Do not heat honey or cook with honey. According to Ayurveda, cooked honey clogs the system and becomes toxic. Most honey you buy in the store has been heated during processing, so check the label closely to make sure you are buying "raw" honey.

3. Do not mix yogurt with sour fruits or melons or mangoes.

4. Don't eat hot and ice-cold foods together (like the favorite—coffee and ice cream). Cold foods or drinks will suppress your digestion, whereas hot foods or drinks will activate it. This creates confusion in the system, disturbs the digestion, and results in formation of ama.

That's it. Deciding not to mix foods can be a bit trouble-some at first, like sorting through the stack of shoes in the clos-et and making some sense out of them. Once those shoes are sorted, you probably find it easier to make quick switches from business shoes to tennis shoes to cross trainers. Your stomach, similarly, likes to be able to know right away which foods to take on at which times.

An Anti-Cancer "Pepto Bismol"

What if you're doing everything right but your digestion still needs a little boost? The drugstore can't really help.—Almost everything there is to help you after you've already got indi-gestion. As we mentioned before, taking a little bit of fresh gin-ger before the meal helps wake up the digestive process. If you're having trouble with your digestion and want to "call out the big guns," take an herbal preparation that really juices up your digestion.

There's a natural preparation you can make that will wake up your digestion without causing any feeling of acid stomach or burning—Pomegranate Seed Chutney. Here's how to make it:

Pomegranate Seed Chutney

Ingredients:
  8 tsp. pomegranate seed powder
  2 tsp. rock salt (or some other type of natural salt)
  ¼ tsp. ground black pepper
  2 tsp. roasted cumin seeds
  ¼ tsp. ground large cardamom seed (this is the large black type, not the small green type)
  15 tsp. fructose
  ½ tsp. lemon juice

Directions:
1. Roast the cumin seeds carefully in a heavy skillet using medium heat. Stir 2 to 3 minutes until they start turning a brownish color, then remove from the heat.

2. Make a powder of all the dry ingredients. You can use a coffee grinder or a small food processor to do this.
3. Mix the lemon juice into the powder.
4. Store the mixture in an airtight container.
5. To use, mix the dry chutney with water or lassi (mentioned earlier in this chapter) to make a thick paste. Eat it with your meals. The serving size is 1 to 2 tsp. per meal.

Note of caution: Don't eat this chutney on an empty stomach, or if you have an acid stomach, or if you are feeling heat in the stomach.

Some well-known herbs for digestion, besides ginger and pomegranate seeds (What, you don't have any in your spice drawer?) are black cumin, black pepper, and the ever-popular tamarind bark.

One preparation has gone to the trouble of tracking down all these ingredients, handling them with loving care (which matters to them), mixing them up in the right proportions, and creating a sizzling synergy that sends a Vedic wake-up call to your system. It's called *Herbal Digest.* Luckily, these tablets have all the ingredients just mentioned. Here's what's in Herbal Digest:

Pomegranate Seeds, Black Cumin, Rock Sugar, Asafoetida, Long Pepper (Catkins), Dried Ginger, Cumin Seeds, Cinnamon, Black Pepper, Rock Salt, Cardamom, and Tamarind Bark.

You could try eating the ingredients separately—a handful of pomegranate seeds, a mouthful of rock sugar. But we don't recommend that approach, and it won't work as well. Herbal Digest has all the ingredients in the right proportions so that they balance each other and bring out the best in each other.

Here's how to take it:

Take one to two tablets of Herbal Digest twice daily, just before lunch and dinner, to increase your appetite. (Take it after meals if your problem is bloating or indigestion.)

The herbs in this formulation can really stimulate your

digestion, and you should find yourself feeling very good as you get more and more of the full value of your food. (For information on how to get the Herbal Digest tablets, see the section "Product Recommendations" at the end of the book.)

Food. Everybody loves it. Nobody can get enough of it. Satisfy yourself one minute, and the next minute you're ready for a fresh plateful of the stuff. Looking for a cancer-fighting ally? You'll find one of the best in dear, adorable food. Grains, dals, fruits, and veggies can turn your body into a veritable fortress against unhealthy invaders. Following a few little cautions will help, such as using a little timing for when you drink your glass of milk. Use a little wisdom in how you eat, and your stomach will do its work better. Short term, a happier stomach means a happier you. Long term, it means a you that is much more likely to prevent the ravages of cancer.

Six

Shake the Sugar Shackles

Sugar. Who can get enough of it? Walk through an airport, and what do you smell?—The sticky, irresistible aroma of Cinnabon sticky buns filling the air. You start to salivate. Your nose takes you to the sugar-covered wonders, a meal in themselves, and you can't resist having just one of the six-inch-in-diameter delights (or two).

Walk past the airport newsstand, and the first display you see—right next to the cash register, for that impulse buy—is the tantalizing candy bar display. Snickers bars. Hershey's milk chocolate bars. Hershey's milk chocolate with almonds. Baby Ruth. Butterfinger. Almond Joy. M & Ms. M & M Peanut. Reese's Peanut Butter Cup. Reese's Pieces. Hershey's kisses.

Walk over to the cooler, and right beside the water are the Eskimo pies. Go into a restaurant, and the dessert menu screams out at you.—Strawberry Cheesecake Supreme. Devil's Food Chocolate Cake. Brownie a la Mode.

Sugar, sugar, sugar. Everybody loves it. Everybody indulges in it. Parents may not give cigarettes to their children, but they give them candy. It's Mother's Day? Give candy to your mother or to your wife. Valentine's Day? Show her you love her with a box of Godiva chocolates. Going to the beach? Walk the boardwalk and eat some cotton candy. Wash it down with a Coke. Sugar. Sugar. Sugar.

Bored while driving? Pull into the truck stop and buy a shrink-wrapped chocolate chip cookie. Buy two, they're big. Have a giant, chug-sized cola along with it. Let the crumbs fall in your lap as you drive a few hours to the next truck stop and the next cookies. Sugar. Sugar. Sugar.

You can't always find a carrot when you want one. Apples can be out of season. If you're dying for some spinach, you can be out of luck sometimes. But you can always get candy. Hard candy. Soft candy. Twirled candy. Stick candy. Caramel candy. Jelly candy. Liquid candy. Real candy. Virtual candy.

Drop back from our earth a few hundred miles and take a close look, and you might think that people are floating not on giant salt water oceans but in a sea of sugar. For birthday parties, people eat chocolate cakes. For Christmas, the sugar starts at Thanksgiving and runs to Martin Luther King Day—peanut brittle, candy canes, ribbon candy, panucci, chocolate fudge, maple fudge...

Sometimes in our cities you could almost suffocate for lack of air. Yet, you can duck into any store or just stop at a stand and buy sugar. It's so commonplace that you can eat it continuously and not even realize it. A few Lifesavers here and there. Some random chocolates from the dish in the show room. An after-dinner mint. A couple teaspoonfuls in your tea. You eat it. You love it. You don't even know it. You're addicted.

The experts say that the average American eats 150 grams of sucrose a day, with other sugars added to it. (Sucrose is the type of sugar you buy at the grocery store.) Granted, 150 grams may not sound like much, because you may not be in the habit of thinking in grams. It's about one-third of a pound, though, and to be honest about it, you probably eat more than that...sometimes in one sitting.

Sugar might seem like one of the few pleasures the Puritan

tradition has left us with. Well, if you're serious about preventing cancer, strike sugar from your list of approved pleasures as well. You need a little, but a little goes a long way. Cancer cells feast on sugar, and rob your other cells of it. However, you can pretty easily solve this addiction, and there's a natural herb that will help you do it.

What's Wrong With It?

What's wrong with having a little innocent sugar now and then anyway? It's an energy booster, isn't it? It makes you happy, and it doesn't hurt anybody. Nobody except a diabetic ever dies from a sugar overdose. You can eat it and nothing else all day, and you'll most likely wake up the next day just fine. And you can do that day after day.

Sugar. One of the biggest problems may just be that it is so ubiquitous, so loved, and so trusted. Everybody eats sugar. Where's the rub?

Tumor Cells Love Sugar

One hint of the potential dangers of sugar is that tumor cells love it. If any tumor cells should happen to be developing in your body, know what they are looking for? Sugar. Obviously, you'd love to starve any cancerous or pre-cancerous cells if you could. You won't do it by eating a Snickers and chasing it with a Mountain Dew.

Cancer cells, it turns out, can't metabolize fat nearly as well as they can glucose. They look for glucose at every turn. (Glucose, which also has the name blood sugar, is what sucrose and all carbohydrates turn into in the body. It's, well, sugar the way your body sees it as it circulates around to the cells.) But cancer cells thrive on glucose. They suck up three to five times as much glucose as normal cells. They're ravenous. They'd kill for it, and they do kill healthy cells by depriving them of the sugar those healthy ones need.

Willing to compete in any underhanded way, these morally bankrupt cancer cells actually secrete stuff that prevents normal cells from taking up the glucose the cancer cells are rabid for. As the normal cells fail to get the energy they need, the person who owns them develops cachexia (loss of skeletal muscle mass) and hyperglycemia (tons of sugar in the blood, because, even though they block the other cells from getting it, the hoggish cancer cells can't eat it all themselves. They just like to know there's plenty of it around, for when they're ready for it). Lots of cancer patients get hyperglycemia, about 60 percent of them.

Some experiments have found that colon cells really thrive on sugar (or, as the scientific articles put it, "sucrose directly affects colon cell proliferation.") And studies have linked sugar to a higher risk of colon cancer. Liver cells (well, mice liver cells in the experiments) grow faster if sugar is around, and sugar in those unfortunate mice assists the development of liver cancer. Mice who have quite a bit of sugar also suffer from more mammary tumors (which could translate into breast cancer in humans) than mice who don't have as much sugar.

And the litany goes on. (Admittedly, sometimes with mice as the evidence, but, hey, scientists do their experiments on mice a lot. The reason for this is because, believe it or not, rodents get a lot of the same diseases humans do, and the course of these diseases is the same in them as it is in us. So, studying mice and rats can give us some potentially valuable information about how our own bodies function. Wild, isn't it?) Mice who have cancer and who have lots of sugar in their diets die sooner than mice with cancer who don't indulge in all the sweets. (Tumors grow faster in the sugar-indulging mice, too.)

Increases Insulin, which Makes Cancer Spread Faster

Know something else sugar does that cancer cells love? It stokes up the insulin in your body. Insulin helps the body use sugar. When there's more sugar in the blood, the body makes more insulin to help handle it. Sugars increase insulin secretion.

Insulin causes cells to reproduce quickly (which isn't what you want in the case of cancer cells). Some studies have found that insulin is a cancer promoter, and have shown that insulin can promote breast cancer (and that *is* in humans).

Also, insulin helps the body form prostaglandin E_2 (which promotes inflammation and helps tumors to spread).

Weakens the Immune System

If the fact that cancer cells love insulin doesn't cause you to pause in midair with that fudge brownie in your hand, think about this. Sugar seems to weaken your immune system. At the cellular level, where cancer happens, the immune system means disease fighters like lymphocytes (white blood cells) and neutrophils (other white blood cells that kill bacteria). When you eat sugar, your body tends to have fewer of those infinitesimal disease fighters. One researcher found that people had 50 percent fewer neutrophils two hours after eating sugar. That's a big drop! And, if fighting disease is your goal, that probably isn't good.

Sugar may also hamper the effectiveness of the neutrophils that you do have. One theory is that the sugar may prevent Vitamin C from entering the neutrophils. When Vitamin C enters the neutrophils, their function improves. However, sugar prevents this from happening. A study has found that, thanks to sugar in the system, cancer cells may grow faster due to decreased functioning of white blood cells.

One scientific article suggests that "most Americans have chronically depressed immune systems." Well, who wants chronic depression of anything? And your immune system, especially, you want in top form. It will do more than anything else to prevent cancer from ever getting a start.

Increases Lactic Acid

As tumor cells gobble up their glucose at a rate three to five times faster than regular cells, they give off extra lactic acid as the natural by-product of their overindulgence. Lactic acid isn't that great to have around. Tumor cells, for one thing, love an acidic environment and grow faster there. Also, lactic acid seems to help the body produce new blood vessels, which cancer loves as it spreads.

Chuck the Chocolate While You're at It

Chocolate is the great sidekick of sugar. Everybody likes to have their sugar in the form of chocolate. Well, you're eliminating sugar already. Chocolate tastes pretty bitter without sugar anyway. While you're limiting your intake of sugar, cut back on the chocolate, too. Your cancer prevention campaign will be the better for the choice.

Fine, But How Do You Get Rid of It?

Boy, does the body ever have a will of its own. "Sugar craving." It can be as irresistible as any of the body's other cravings. You can begin to cut back on your intake of sugar just by having the intention to do so. Try having dessert with just one meal a day (lunch) instead of all three. Try having a piece of fruit for a snack instead of a chocolate éclair. Drink bottled water instead of soda. Gradually recondition yourself. (Want to know how much sugar is in a 12 ounce can of soda? Ten teaspoons. Really. We have the reference on it.)

It can work, but the body can be pretty insistent in its cravings. Few among us can keep from giving in to the sugar urges, especially if nobody is watching and (as is the case from the gas station to the supermarket to the restaurant to the neighborhood news stand) the temptation is present. "I'll just have one square of a chocolate bar," we tell ourselves, and, before we know it, the six-pack of chocolate bars in the cupboard is history.

You can give your body a little assist. Here's an Ayurvedic secret. Try a little *Gymnema sylvestre*. This gentle herb, usually known by just its first name, gymnema, is the "sugar stomper outer." It works on more than one front, too. First of all, gymnema takes away the taste of sugar. It does. Take a little bit, then put some sugar on your tongue. Most people say the same thing.—"It tastes like sand." Gymnema's active ingredient is "gymnemic acid," and the molecules in it look to the body like sugar molecules. The molecules fill the receptor locations on your taste buds, so, when a little glucose comes along, there's "no one home" (i.e. no taste buds) to receive it. You don't taste the sweetness. As a bonus, gymnema takes away the taste of bitter as well, so chocolate won't have its usual allure for you either.

When it gets into your small intestine, the gymnemic acid also does a little imposter number. It fills up the receptor locations for sugar in the intestine, preventing sugar from using them instead. Sugar passes out of the body instead of into the blood stream. Your blood sugar heads in the right direction, namely down.

Western researchers have begun to document the beneficial effects of gymnema but, of course, they don't fully understand how to use it properly. (OK, they're clueless, but how would it sound for us to say that? They have absolutely no idea of the right use of gymnema and are as likely to have you sucking it all day long or eating potent extracts of it as they are to somehow luckily strike on the right dosage.) Here is an admission from one discussion of gymnema in Western science: "The most appropriate dose is unknown…A minimum and maximum effective and safe dose is unknown."

What Western medicine doesn't know about gymnema, though, Ayurvedic medicine had known for a few thousand generations. One good place to get the right dose of gymnema in the right combination with other herbs is from *Be Trim* tea. Just have a cup of this tea two or three times a day, and your body won't have that irresistible craving for "just a couple of bonbons, maybe a few mints."

When you're ready for dessert following a meal, first have two or three fresh dates. (Organic Medjool dates are so good they can take your mind completely off hot fudge sundaes for the moment.) Have some other dried fruits, if you like. The brain needs some sugar, so you shouldn't try to eliminate all sugar from your diet.

Once you've had some sweets, take the Be Trim tea.

Sit quietly for five minutes following your meal, then easily resume activity.

Here's what's in the Be Trim tea:

Mint Leaf, Fennel Seed, Indian Kino, Gymnema Sylvestre, Manjista, Cinnamon Stick, Cardamom, Black Pepper, Long Pepper, Turmeric Root, Rose Petal, Licorice Root.

The tea will help you develop a little moral strength, enough to resist that piece of chocolate cake with strawberries. (Just have the strawberries instead.) For information on how to get the Be Trim tea, see the section "Product Recommendations" at the end of the book.

Sugar, sugar, sugar. Nobody thinks of it as a bad word. Nobody thinks of it as a bad substance. Maybe a few health extremists have attacked it here and there, but with about as much success as enemies of video games and television. No appreciable success. Sugar is fun, and what can it hurt?

Well, it can feed cells that want to become cancerous. Also, it can really depress your immune system, and, if you think about it, your immune system does a lot more every day than fight against cancer. It fights against everything—colds, flu, any kind of bacteria, virus, or toxin that might go swimming around in your body. You probably want to keep it as strong as you possibly can.

You may need a little assist in your fight against sugar addiction, of course. You're only human. Gymnema can do that for you. Have a little gymnema, and sugar becomes as tasteless as some of the late-night TV humor.

Seven

Self-Administer Interleukin-2

What is it in our society? You read all the time about jet-setting CEOs who work 80-hour weeks to get where they are. You never read about top CEOs who *sleep* 56-hour weeks. You read about ballplayers who tell us the secret to their 5 million dollar bonuses.—They worked tirelessly, while the competition was apparently just goofing off. You don't hear that they rest diligently.

Everywhere you turn, society seems to encourage activity while running roughshod over sleep. Redeye flights from LA to NY and vice versa can't keep up with the demand.—People ride a plane all night, work on the plane instead of sleeping, and then go directly to a meeting on Monday morning. Such cavalier dismissing of sleep is supposed to make them into star performers.

Yet, creativity and clarity of mind are the key to success. Plenty of evidence points to lost productivity in the workplace because of lack of sleep in the employees. According to an estimate from the National Sleep Foundation, sleepiness is costing us $18 billion a year in lost productivity. Freshness is vital, and we *almost* know it, but so far the driving message to society seems to be the incorrect "Drive yourself. Drive. Drive. Drive. Work. Work. Work. Sleep only when you finally collapse from fatigue, and then only fitfully. Then wake up and work."

In point of fact, sleep is as potent as anything you can do for being successful in your work. It's also a great cancer preventative. Slumber may be *the* most potent thing you can do for your health because of the astonishing restorative and reviving power the body unleashes when you are basically doing nothing. Nothing at all. "You" are not even there. Your body takes care of itself, and it does a pretty fine job of it without you getting in the way.

Your Anti-Cancer Chemo Factory

How does the passivity, the outright surrender of sleep help to prevent cancer? Many ways. Science has begun to document some.

Sleep comes on thanks to small molecules called cytokines that help cells talk to each other. They are the kind of chemical components in the body that you want to keep in balance if you want to keep your cells happy and your DNA alert and not confused. Cytokines build up in your body in response to the toxins that build up as you fatigue during the day. (Their job gets harder, so there are more of them.) One of the most famous of them is Interleukin-2.

Interleukin-2 is a known anti-cancer commando, well-appreciated enough that medicine in fact administers Interleukin-2 treatments to those fighting cancer. Talk about expediters. This particular cytokine is like an advance spy who tells friendly guns exactly where to fire. The body's firepower against cancerous tendencies are the white blood cells. During sleep, white blood cells go surging around the body looking for pathogens of any sort and wiping them out. Some of the cells joining in the nightly anti-toxin crusade have names as fearsome as their activity—T cells (think Tasmanian devil) and, even better named, Natural Killer cells (NK cells).

How does the Interleukin-2 help these friendly marauders?

It attaches to errant cells (such as cancer cells) and guides cancer-destroying white blood cells directly to them.

What does sleep have to do with it? The Interleukin-2 increases significantly during sleep.You can think of sleep as a self-administered Interleukin-2 treatment, where the self-manufactured cytokine is perfectly tuned to the needs of your body and the receptivity of your own white blood cells. It is a perfect member of the anti-cancer team, because your body tailors it specifically for the task at hand.

There are numerous cytokines besides the widely publicized Interleukin-2, of course, and plenty of chemical warriors that are not cytokines but enzymes or other substances. Interferon is an anti-cancer warrior you may have heard of.The FDA has approved it for treating a certain type of leukemia and some other diseases. Science is beginning to identify cytokines and how they work. Of course, the body already knows all of them and how they work, and it manufactures them all for you …particularly if you happen to let the body do its thing by sleeping.

Participating in the great cancer prevention war as you sleep are such other players as the currently-in-vogue melatonin and prolactin.The hormone melatonin helps to bring on sleep. During actual sleep, the melatonin increases. One of its benefits is to increase your cytokines like interferon and interleukin-2. Also, melatonin is itself a great free-radical fighter. At the deepest sleep, your body also secretes the hormone prolactin, which gets your white blood cells doing an even better "search-and-destroy" job on toxins sneaking around in your body and trying to confuse the DNA.

Another cytokine has earned the name tumor necrosis factor (TNF) because scientists have found that it caused at least one type of cancer to die. (Necrosis is a scientific term for death.) TNF, it's worth noting, increases tenfold during sleep.

You can, it's true, purchase Interleukin-2 therapy and treatments with other interleukins, with interferon, and with other cytokines. Studies, for instance, have found that Interleukin-2 may have some effectiveness against ovarian cancer and other research is looking at its usefulness for fighting melanoma as well as breast and prostate cancers.

However, if you wait to purchase these substances and use them as prescribed pharmaceuticals, you run all kinds of risks. First of all, you may not even realize you need them until quite late in the battle against cancer…after the cancer has already started. Besides, by having scientists apply the treatments, you're relying on limited human intelligence to decide which chemicals to apply, in what quantities, and for how long. Side effects are inevitable. Have the body decide during sleep which ones to put into action, and the right choices are automatic.

Vedic medicine has long had its own language for the chemicals that build up during sleep and for the toxins that get eliminated. If you don't sleep well, you build up ama in the body—that whitish substance that clogs the channels in the body and causes ill health. If you do sleep well, you build nice quantities of ojas, the vital life force that literally strengthens the underlying basis of DNA—pure consciousness. The better you sleep, the more ama you clean out and the more ojas you produce.

Getting the Factory Working

Deciding to sleep is probably the biggest obstacle to proper rest these days. People feel guilty about sleeping. "I should be working until midnight or beyond," we think. "Otherwise, how am I going to get in the 80 hours this week it takes to become a millionaire CEO with a golden parachute?" (Those 80-hour weeks, when you think about it, include some really long meals, and some meetings with a lot of daydreaming going on.)

Suppose you have decided you want to sleep. Having crossed the biggest hurdle, you're ready to get real results. But not everybody finds good sleep easy to come by. And, the better the quality of your sleep, the more powerful the anti-cancer effect. So here are some guidelines to help you get the proper slumber you need.

Sleep at Night ("Quit Your Night Job.")

The best time to sleep is at night. Such advice might seem like the baldest common sense. In our modern world, though, we have to get right back to the basic basics; because many of us get so turned around in our artificially lighted worlds that at times we're not even sure whether it is day or night.

Even if we lose our rhythms, though, nature keeps its own rhythms intact. The sun rises at a certain time, follows a cycle throughout the day, and sets at a certain time. The more you attune your body's rhythms to nature's rhythms, the more you gain strength and eliminate weakness.

Ayurveda recommends that you get to sleep before 10 PM. The hours from 6 to 10 PM are a naturally drowsy time, beneficial to falling asleep easily. The hours from 10 PM to 2 AM—when many are in the habit of going to bed following the Late Show—are not as beneficial for falling asleep. Certain systems in the body are active at that time—systems of digestion and purification. If you get to sleep during the drowsy time and hand your body over to your night crew, that crew does the best job of cleaning out impurities while strengthening immunity with substances like Interleukin-2.

Don't Sleep During the Day

This advice is a corollary of the previous advice. Sleep, yes, is good. Like everything, there is a time and place for it. During the hot summer months a little daytime siesta is good. If you're sick, sleep any time. That's good. For the most part, though, sleep during the day aggravates certain tendencies toward sluggishness and headache. Sleep at night.

Try a Little Bedtime Tryptophan

How do you sleep right? If you like to know you're consuming a pharmaceutical and not just ordinary food (and who among us doesn't like the medicinal sound of real drugs), here's a way to get yourself to sleep at night. Try a little of the essential amino acid tryptophan.

Tryptophan helps your body produce the neurotransmitter serotonin, which facilitates sleep. Tryptophan stabilizes moods, promotes sleep, and helps ease the effects of stress. It seems to help fight depression. It helps build rich, red blood; is good for your hair; and helps your skin, too. Tryptophan aids in digestion and helps the body use the B vitamins better (vitamins that help build healthy cells, particularly nerve cells).

You can't buy it as an extract, though. The government pulled it off the market in 1989, because a contaminated batch had hit the streets. But, if you want to take this sleep inducer, there's a safe, natural way to do it. Drink some warm milk before bed. (As we mentioned before, the reason for heating the milk is because it's easier to digest that way.)

You can try adding some innocent poppy seeds to your diet, too. Having a few on your bagel will have a gentle relaxing effect and help prepare you for your sleep later on.

Really want to treat yourself with some nighttime tryptophan? Go all out with a Date Milk Shake. Here's how to make one:

Date Milk Shake

Ingredients:

> 4–5 whole dates (Medjool variety or similar is best. They're sweet and rich.)
> 1 cup whole organic milk (not homogenized is better)
> 2 pinches cinnamon powder

Directions:

1. Boil the milk and let it foam once, then turn off the heat.
2. Put the milk, dates (don't forget to remove the pits), and cinnamon in a blender, and blend until the dates are finely ground.
3. In the winter, serve it warm. In the summer, serve it at room temperature or even slightly cooler (but not cold).

Nothing is working? Sometimes the mind is just too jazzed. Sleep won't come, or if it does, it won't stay for long. You don't have to reach for the sleeping pills. You can call in the services of a gentle food supplement. We recommend a preparation called *Blissful Sleep*. These tablets have a little Indian Valerian Root in them, which residents of the Eastern nation have long known has a soothing effect. Muskroot is in there, and that will calm a person down. Winter Cherry helps balance your mind and emotions. It's those imbalances that keep you awake, so balancing is good. Here's everything that's in the Blissful Sleep tablets, put together with synergy in mind:

Indian Valerian Root Extract, Rose Petals, Muskroot (Nardostachys Jatamansi), Heart-Leaved Moonseed (Guduchi), Winter Cherry (Ashwagandha), Trikatu [consisting of Black Pepper, Long Pepper (Pippali), Ginger], Pearl Bhasma, Aloeweed (Shankapushpi), and Licorice Root.

Take one to two tablets just before bedtime at night with a bit of natural sugar and warm milk or water. To see where to get it, check the section "Product Recommendations" at the end of the book.

Don't Read in Bed

It's easy to think that it's relaxing to read in bed for a while before turning off the light. Even more popular, and also not recommended, is watching television in bed before going to sleep. Reading and watching TV keep your mind active at a time when you want it to settle down completely. It's also best not to bring any work-related material into your bedroom. Don't have your PC in there. Don't bring in manila folders from work. Don't pile up your textbooks in the bedroom. Bedrooms are for sleeping, and they work best if you let them focus on their primary purpose.

Finish Your Evening Meal Two to Three Hours Before Going to Bed

Eating gets your digestion working. It wakes up that digestive fire we've mentioned before—namely, enzymes that are fiery in nature. For sleep, though, you want cooling effects. It's best if you can finish eating two to three hours before you go to bed.

Also, for that evening meal, don't go heavy on the chilis and hot sauce. Avoid spicy foods at that time, for the same reason as just mentioned—keeping your physiology cool.

As for the modern craze to have a cup of Starbuck's coffee in your hand all the time, gradually wean yourself from that attachment. Any stimulant has the contrasting effect with sleep. Even alcohol, though seemingly relaxing, is actually a stimulant and won't help you sleep.

Get Relaxed

In the spirit of being easy and relaxed as you go to sleep, here are a couple more pointers. Wear comfortable clothing to bed. Natural fibers are best, especially cotton. Keep the bedroom dark. Light in the bedroom fools your body into thinking it's not really nighttime, and it doesn't produce as many of the beneficial nighttime chemicals as it otherwise would. If you want to get into the mood for a good sleep, slide into a warm bath before bed. You can also massage the soles of your feet with coconut oil before bed. And it's good to practice the ultimate relaxation technique twice daily—*Transcendental Meditation (TM)*. This technique has been studied and shown to improve sleep in those who practice it.

Following a Good Routine Around the Clock

Sleep starts when you wake up. Well, that's an intentional paradox, but the best way to be ready to sleep well at night is to prepare yourself for sleep all day long by staying in balance and keeping a healthy routine. Here is a good routine to follow:

Get to Bed on Time (Before 10 PM)

This is the key to everything else. Somehow persuade yourself to do this. Start getting ready earlier and douse the lights by 10. Getting to bed at 9 is even better, actually, but 10 is curfew time for sure.

Wake Up Early

You'll naturally wake up early anyway if you get to bed by 10pm. By 6am you'll have had 8 hours of nourishing sleep.

Practice Transcendental Meditation

The point of all anti-cancer techniques is to keep the cells of the body aware of themselves and not have them lapsing into confusion. During the transcending of Transcendental Meditation, both your mind and your cells become alert. Meditation heightens cell intelligence. Meditation in the early morning primes your physiology for a focused and lively day of activity.

Eat a Good Breakfast with Stewed Apple, Fiber

Get your digestion working for you right away with a stewed apple. Have a little cereal, too, or something rich in fiber (which, as mentioned in Chapter 2, is great for strengthening your digestion and doing other things like keeping your blood sugar steady).

Take a Morning Walk

This Vedic technique is the coming fashion in the health-conscious set. The walk gets your blood circulating, which brings cytokines, neuropeptides, and multiple nourishing and cancer-fighting substances to parts of the body that just get neglected during normal blood circulation.

Also, if you catch the morning as it is just waking up, you have a wonderful experience of blending with the birds, the sun, and nature-as-a-whole as it rises into life. You enjoy a surge of fresh life along with your surroundings. (A sunrise walk is also an antidote to depression.)

Work, Play, or Study

Work isn't bad; just overwork is bad. In fact, a dynamic life is valuable in preventing cancer.

Eat Lunch on Time

Around noontime, the digestion is primed for action. It is ready for the foods you'll introduce. If you don't satisfy it then, the digestive ability fades a bit. Besides, some imbalances may come up when the body can't find the food it wants to satisfy itself. Appetites may begin to go out of whack.

Work, Play, or Study

As in the morning, dynamic activity is good.

Meditate

You should balance your activity with rest. Meditation in the late afternoon relieves you of the stresses accumulated during the day, and relaxes you so you can fully enjoy your low-key evening activities.

Eat a Light Dinner Three Hours Before Bed

Remember, nothing too spicy. In case you weren't counting, this would be the third meal of the day. That's the optimum number. Eat three meals a day. A light snack three hours after lunch is all right, too.

Don't Work at Night

Professional athletes don't have a choice. Their games sometimes get scheduled at night. They retire early, though, and can go onto a normal schedule. The rest of us may feel we have no choice but to work at night either. Find ways out of it, though. You'll more than make up for the lost time with your alertness and productivity the next day.

Spend the evening with your family or friends, and don't be shy to spend other times with your family as well. Meal times make sense for a little family fun.

Have a Little Tryptophan, and Get to Bed Before 10 PM

Have some warm milk. Complete the cycle where you began, and repeat it the next day. Regular routine is a pillar of

Ayurveda, one of the most powerful things you can do to keep yourself cancer free.

To some degree, in our society, we just have it backwards, then. We think that life is only about being awake, only about working. So we prop our eyelids open and work until we drop. Such a life style is a cancer breeding ground. Those night-janitor cytokines don't get a chance to do their work properly, because the "building" they're trying to clean (the body) is never at rest and is generating impurities even as they try to clean them out. Proper sleep, though, is a powerful chemical war against cancerous tendencies in your body. It means that cancer has a heck of a time ever getting started.

❧ Eight

"Just Detox, Ma'am, Just Detox"

"Detox." Usually, when you hear the term at all in ordinary life, you hear it as a euphemism for "drying out" from an alcohol or drug addiction. "Detoxification" is the full term clinicians use and, we must admit, it sounds imposing, off-putting, a little bit ugly…as in, "whatever *detox* is, I don't want anything to do with it." People don't even want to think about something from the elimination end of the spectrum. However, you can actually detoxify yourself while rather enjoying yourself at the same time. You don't even really have to think of it as purification, just as airing out your cells a little bit as you enjoy yourself. A nice, easy 20-minute walk is a great form of detox. If you don't want to read this whole chapter, just make a little walking part of your routine. You'll be missing some really fun techniques if you skip this chapter, though, and some more focused, effective techniques than just random walking around. Given that toxins are cancer-causers, detox is a natural cancer preventer. This chapter shows how you can nicely cleanse your cells each day without a lot of unnecessary effort.

"Detox" and Cancer?

What, after all, causes cancer in the first place? Some tiny little thing in the tiny little cell causes the DNA to forget itself and become confused. The tiny little thing can take many different forms—from unwanted chemicals to pesky free radicals—but this much is sure about them.... they don't belong where they are, hanging around the DNA, annoying it, and possibly driving it to distraction. Toxins cause cancer.

Would a list of toxins make this reasoning more persuasive? Here are some of the gazillion toxins human cells are swimming around in every day:

- Industrial toxins (you know, like lead, arsenic, DDT, and aluminum)
- Pollution from water (containing stuff like gasoline solvents, not to mention chlorine and fluoride)
- Nicotine, carbon monoxide, and other harmful toxins from smoking
- Bovine growth hormone, fed to your favorite cows and present in your milk unless you're one of the few who refuse to buy milk containing BGH
- Steroids, such as cortisone steroids used in cattle
- Vaccines, which, nice as they are, have foreign RNA/DNA fragments, live viruses, aluminum, mercury, formalin, formaldehyde, and MSG
- Parasites (which live in the intestine, blood, lymph, heart, liver, gallbladder, pancreas, spleen, eyes, brain ...and give off—you guessed it—toxins)
- Alcohol (which, face it, ain't natural, and does things like suppress your cancer-fighting Natural Killer cells and stress your liver)
- Caffeine (not just from coffee, of course, but from tea, colas, and chocolate. It can damage the DNA)
- Food additives (BHA, BHT, sulfites, nitrites, aspartame and nitrofurans. The FDA likes them OK, but your cells probably aren't that fond of them.)
- Mercury (from your dental fillings)

It's discouraging, as we mentioned. No wonder nobody wants to think about detox. The enemy (all those toxins) is flooding the body. Who has any chance against it?

The body, of course, is wondrous. It can cleanse itself incredibly well. Still, it likes some assistance if you can provide it. It would be nice if you could, say, filter the cell to take out whatever impurities might be trying to take up residence there. But you can't really filter your cells like that. What you can do is create the conditions where the body purifies itself. (Even alcohol detox isn't really some formal process so much as avoiding the impurity for a while to allow the body to restore itself, which it willingly does given half a chance.) If the cell is strong enough, impurities won't bother it. So, you can help the cell along in its purification regimen with the gentle cell-awakening techniques we discuss in this chapter.

From the point of view of preventing cancer, detox would be as strong a candidate as anything for creating the conditions where cancer just could not arise. With no poisons around to corrupt the cell, what could go wrong? And detox, as its name suggests, drives off toxins (or, in other words, gets rid of poisons).

Putting the X in Detox—X...ercise

If exercise was all you had to do to detoxify yourself, people might be receptive to the idea. In fact, exercise does do a great deal to flush out impurities in the body.

Everyone in authority these days seems to extol the glories of exercise. Here are some examples:

- Heart physicians have their patients on treadmills almost the moment they complete their bypass operations. Exercise makes your heart muscle stronger and lowers the "bad" cholesterol (LDL: low-density lipoprotein).
- Exercise helps lower blood pressure. It also helps you lose weight, which further helps lower blood pressure, a powerful tandem of treatments for lengthening your life.

- Movement is good for preventing arthritis and for combating it.
- Physicians recommend exercise as a way to combat diabetes. Studies have found that somehow exercise improves your ability to use insulin. (If you use insulin well, you digest sugar better, and you help lessen your chances of getting diabetes and, by the way, cancer.)
- Nothing, except maybe controlled diet, seems to match exercise for fighting obesity. In the case of obesity, exercise means swapping fat (which is bad) for muscle (which is good). Exercise also helps you digest foods well so that they don't turn into fat in the first place.

And the beat goes on. You hear recommendations for exercise so much these days that you have to wonder why so few people seem to be listening. You can't walk into a department store without bumping into the latest in treadmills and "wondrous," life-saving exercise devices. Flip the pages of your favorite magazine, and exercise aids jump out at you (along with ads for the drugs that will help you if you think it's too late for exercise). Flip the channels on the TV and you get the same result, particularly when you land on those infomercials for cool, twisted metal devices that will make you look as beautiful as the flat-stomached emcee for the show. Exercise.—Everybody knows about it; nobody does it.

How does exercise help purify the body? When you exercise, your heart pumps faster. That increased pumping increases blood flow to the lungs, where the blood picks up fresh oxygen. Thus enriched, the pumped blood goes rushing off to parts of the body that otherwise see only pedestrian blood flow (or little blood flow at all). The fresh, healthy blood flows to the brain, which gets both nourished and cleansed. It flows to your arms, your fingers, your knees, your stomach, your colon, your liver, your feet. It bathes all those tissues with fresh oxygen, the great cleaning lady of the cell.

Now, plenty of studies affirm that exercise is beneficial at the structural level as well as the cellular level of the body. People who exercise have less risk of colon cancer than those who don't, at least in part because the exercise helps them push food through the bowel faster. Exercise seems to decrease the risk of breast cancer, and some studies suggest that the reason may be that exercise causes you to produce less estrogen. In addition, exercise improves your mood by releasing chemicals in the brain, such as every runner's favorite—endorphins. (Exercise has some of the same anti-cancer benefits as positive behavior, which we discuss in Chapter 9.)

There's exercise, of course, and then there's intelligent exercise. You can hurt yourself by exercising too much, exercising in the wrong ways, or exercising at the wrong times. If you follow a few Vedic guidelines in your exercise, you can enliven cell intelligence and purification without doing yourself damage.

Here are some guidelines from Maharishi Vedic Medicine:

1. Exercise to about 50 percent of your capacity. ("No pain, no gain" is not a Vedic principle. In fact, when you feel discomfort, ease off.)
2. Exercise every day. (You can afford to do that with moderate exercise like this, because your body doesn't need a day here and there to recover. You aren't straining it in the first place.)
3. Don't exercise on a full stomach. Wait two hours after eating a full meal, one hour after a light meal. (The best hours for exercise are 6 a.m. to 10 a.m.) There are a few other times when exercising should mean "exercising restraint"—i.e. not exercising. Women experiencing their monthly periods should pass up their daily jog, or any other strenuous exercise. Also, anyone suffering from an acute illness should forget about exercising. The body needs its resources for fighting the illness, not for increasing your metabolism as you exercise.
4. Don't strain when you exercise. (Breathe through the nose. If you find yourself breathing through the mouth, ease off. You'll develop stamina over time.)

If four guidelines are too many for your exercise routine, just follow this one.—Take it easy.

Exercise, then, is detoxifying. Western tradition doesn't know a whole lot about how to maximize the purifying effects of exercise. The Vedic tradition, though, has raised exercise to a fine art that gets maximum detoxifying benefit with the least effort on your part.

Smart Exercise—Yoga

Yoga, as it is popularly termed, has become almost as much a part of our popular culture as cell phones, SUVs, and surfing the Web. Everybody likes yoga these days. "Yoga is a particularly health-enhancing form of exercise," says Candace B. Pert, Ph.D., in her book *Molecules of Emotion.* Yoga, the Sanskrit term for "union," in fact has as its objective to enhance health. Yoga refers to the union of the mind with the cosmic intelligence. Through the practice of yoga, the individual mind gains the state of cosmic intelligence, which is the highest state of evolution.

In this section, we are talking about a specific form of yoga known as *Hatha yoga.* Hatha yoga is the process of establishing perfect physical, mental, emotional, and psychic equilibrium by manipulating the energies of the body. The system of Hatha yoga was designed to transform the physical elements of the body, so they can receive and transmit a much subtler and more powerful energy. This system uses different physical postures, called *asanas,* to achieve this goal. Classes that teach these postures are widely available these days.

Asanas, you might say, are the essence of exercise. They don't replace exercise—they're just a lot smarter. About half an hour a day of brisk but comfortable walking is a good idea; this type of exercise increases blood flow, albeit in pretty much a hit-or-miss fashion. Asanas send blood flowing to particular places in a tactical way. They bring blood flow to particular parts of the body—often parts that are rarely used. A shoulder stand, for instance, gets blood flowing the opposite way from its usual course. (A little "reversing the flow" can be quite refreshing.)

In general, asanas help reduce stress in the body. They sooth the muscles and soften blocks of stress that have been accumulating over a lifetime. There are scores of asanas to choose from. This next section presents a few that will benefit your physiology in general.

Yoga Asanas (Postures)

Important Points

- These postures should be done for about ten minutes either in the morning or in the evening.
- The postures should be done before eating.
- If you've already eaten, wait one hour after a light breakfast, two hours after a regular meal, or 30 minutes after drinking any liquids before doing the postures.
- Wear loose, comfortable clothing.
- Don't strain while doing the postures. Take it easy.

A. Toning Up of the Body

This is a two-minute tone-up of the heart and blood vessels. It involves pressing the blood gently towards the heart.

1. Sit crossed-legged. Place your hands on the top of your head and gradually press and release, moving your hands down your face and neck to your heart. During the pressing and releasing, your hands should not lose contact with your body.
2. Place your hands on the top of your head and gradually press and release, moving your hands down over the back of your neck, then coming around front to your heart.
3. Grasp the fingertips of your right hand with your left hand (palm of left hand should be facing down) and gradually move up your arm, pressing and releasing, moving up to your shoulder and down to your heart.
4. Grasp the fingertips of your right hand with your left hand (palm of left hand should be facing up) and gradually move up your arm, pressing and releasing, moving up to your shoulder and down to your heart.

5. Repeat movements 3 and 4, grasping your left hand with your right hand.

6. Place both hands on your abdomen with the tips of your middle fingers meeting horizontally at your navel. Move up to your heart gradually, pressing and releasing as you go.

7. With both hands press and release your mid-back and ribs up toward your heart as far as you can reach; then follow the ribs around to the front of your chest.

8. Grasp the top of your toes on your right foot with your right hand and the sole of your foot with your left hand and move up your foot and leg, pressing and releasing, moving up to the thigh, then the waist, then to the heart.

9. Repeat movement 8 with the left foot.

10. Lie on your back, draw your knees up toward your chest, and clasp your hands around your legs. Raise your head slightly.

11. Roll to the far right, then roll to the far left, repeating five times in each direction; then slowly release your knees and straighten your legs and arms, laying flat on the floor and relaxing completely.

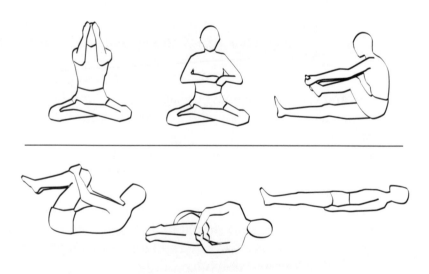

B. Seat Posture

Kneel, sitting on the flats of your feet, heels apart, big toes crossed. Place your hands in your lap with your right hand on top of your left hand, palms up. Hold your head, neck, and spine in a straight line, for 5 seconds. Raise your body up, with your feet, shins, and knees still on the floor, then sit back down as before. Repeat one to three times.

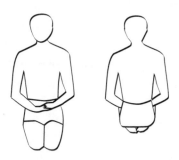

Effect:

Strengthens the pelvic region, removes tension from the knees and ankles, and builds a strong foundation for the base of the back. It also produces many other healthy benefits in the subtle regions of your nervous system.

C. Head Over Knee Posture

1. Sit and stretch your right leg (for men) or your left leg (for women).
2. Bend the other leg, bringing your heel into your abdomen.
3. Bend forward and grasp the center of your right (or left) foot with both hands, arms stretched.
4. Touch your forehead to your knee.
5. Hold for 5 to 15 seconds.
6. Repeat with your other leg.
7. Repeat this sequence one to three times.

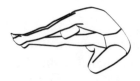

Effect:
   Strengthens and relaxes the spine and abdominal organs.

D. Plough and Half Shoulder Stand Posture

1. Lie on your back with your arms at your sides.
2. Keeping your legs straight, slowly raise them up and hold them slightly past the vertical position; as your hips rise off the floor, support them with your hands. Hold this position for 30 seconds.
3. Keeping your legs straight, slowly lower them over your head until your toes touch the floor. At the same time, straighten your arms and place them on the floor, palms down.
4. Cross your arms around the top of your head and hold for five seconds.
5. Slowly unfold your arms and straighten them out again, palms down, as before.
6. Slowly raise your legs back up over your head and hold them in the same half-vertical position as before, supporting your hips with your hands.
7. Slowly lower your legs to the floor, with your arms at your sides.
8. Repeat one to three times.

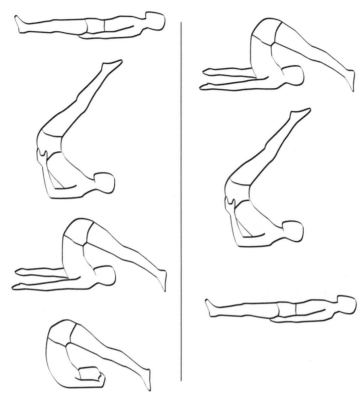

Effect:

Strengthens and relaxes the neck glands (thyroid), back, neck, shoulders, liver, and spleen, removes excess fat and fatigue, improves circulation in the head, improves the eyes and hair, relieves mental fatigue, softens the whole body, and aids in the performance of other postures.

E. Cobra Posture

1. Lie face down with your forehead on the floor and place your palms on the floor beside your shoulders.
2. Slowly raise your head and chest until your back is lifted to the middle part of your backbone. Hold for 10 to 15 seconds.
3. Lower your chest and head to the original position and relax completely.
4. Repeat one to three times.

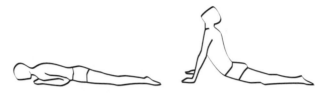

Effect:

Strengthens and relaxes the back muscles, and relieves uterine and ovarian irregularities.

F. Locust Posture

1. Lie face down with your chin resting gently on the floor.
2. Place your arms straight out by your sides, palms up.
3. Raise your legs, keeping them as straight as possible. Hold for a few seconds.
4. Slowly lower your legs back to the floor.
5. Repeat one to three times.

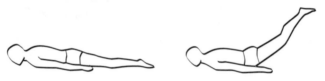

Note:

If it is too difficult to raise your legs in the beginning of practice, place your hands underneath your thighs with your palms touching your thighs. This will support your back while you are raising your legs.

Effect:

Strengthens the lumbar region of the back, and relieves uterine and ovarian irregularities.

G. Twist Posture

1. Sit with your right leg on the floor, bent so your foot rests on its side near your left hip.
2. Cross your left leg over your right leg, and place your left foot flat on the floor to the right of your right knee.
3. Twist your trunk to the left and place your right arm

against the left side of your left leg, and grab the left side of your left ankle with your right hand.

4. Place your left hand on the floor behind your back, palm down.
5. Twist your head and trunk to the left as far as comfortably possible.
6. Hold for ten seconds.
7. Repeat with your other leg.

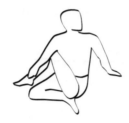

Effect:

   Improves circulation in the liver, spleen, neck, and shoulders.

H. Hand and Foot Pose

1. Stand straight with your feet together and arms at your side.
2. Bend at the waist and touch your toes with your fingers.
3. Touch your forehead to your knees or slightly above them.
4. Hold for five seconds.
5. Stand up straight.
6. Repeat one to three times.

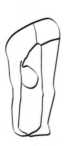

Effect:

Strengthens and improves the internal functioning of the abdominal region and the spinal column, increases digestive secretions, and improves the digestive system, blood circulation in the upper part of the body, and sensory perception.

I. Lying Down Posture

Lie down on your back with your arms at your sides and relax completely for a minute or two, keeping the mind and body loose.

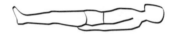

Effect:

This posture allows your body to assimilate the benefits of all the postures you have just finished.

Something as popular as yoga is likely to attract a good deal of scientific research, and in fact, yoga asanas have done just that. Studies have found, for instance, that asanas reduce your serum cholesterol level (cholesterol can clog your blood vessels). Other studies have found reduced blood sugar level (in the morning before eating breakfast), again indicating success against a carcinogen—namely sugar. Studies have found beneficial changes in enzymes. They've found improved mental functioning, too, such as reduced neuroticism and decreased mental fatigue.

If exercise is good, then targeted exercise like the Yoga asanas is particularly good for cancer prevention.

Exercise Essence—Vedic Breathing

Exercise doesn't have to mean running, throwing a football, rolling around, pummeling a punching bag, repeatedly raising and lowering a barbell, walking on a treadmill, or any of what people normally refer to as exercise. It *can* be those things, but the Vedic tradition has forms of exercise even more quietly powerful than the asanas described in the previous section—effective forms of exercise, without harmful side effects like those you can get from running too much or lifting too many barbells.

You can perform a breathing exercise, called *pranayama*, that works with the breath to settle, balance, and refresh (i.e. detoxify) your whole body. Prana is the vital life force and pranayama is the process by which this vital force is increased. It is a technique through which the quantity of prana is raised to a higher energy level. Pranayama is practiced in order to understand and control the vital life force in the body. Breathing is a direct means of absorbing prana and the manner in which we breathe sets off pranic vibrations that influence our entire being. It awakens your inner awareness in your body.

It may be surprising to think you can have such a large effect by doing so little—just some regulated breathing. Western scientific studies have documented some of the good effects of pranayama, such as reduced bronchial asthma attacks. Studies have also found that pranayama creates accelerated adrenocortical functions (and those functions, controlling the body's enzymes, are good in preventing cancer).

Pranayama is the ancient breathing technique for enriching oxygen flow to the brain. According to Vedic tradition, the nose is the gateway to the brain. Pranayama, of course, works through the nose. And it is the brain, above all, that you want to nourish when you exercise. Nourishing the brain, the main switchboard of the body, automatically nourishes the rest of the body as well.

This technique, like asanas, you don't have to practice for a long time. In fact, a little goes a long way.—Five minutes twice a day is good, once in the morning (before meditation if you practice meditation) and once in the evening (again, before meditation, if, you know, you're a meditator).

Here's how to do it:

Pranayama (Breathing Exercise)

1. Sit in a comfortable position.
2. Breathe in through both nostrils.
3. Use your right thumb to close your right nostril and breathe out through your left nostril, slowly and completely.
4. Breathe in slowly and completely through your left nostril, then close your left nostril with the ring and middle fingers of your right hand while opening your right nostril to breathe out. Breathe out slowly and completely through your right nostril.
5. Breathe in again through your right nostril, then repeat steps 3 through 5 for five to ten minutes.

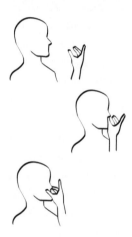

Effect:

Strengthens the lungs and heart, improves digestion, purifies the nervous system, and conserves energy.

That's it. Seems like there ought to be more to it, but there isn't. Breathing purifies the body anyway. This controlled, Vedic breathing purifies it in a focused way.

This little bit of slightly regulated breathing balances your two nervous systems—the parasympathetic and sympathetic. They tend to have opposite effects. The sympathetic nervous system decreases the activity of your salivary glands. The parasympathetic increases it. The sympathetic one raises the heart rate; the other one slows it down. Both systems are regulated by the hypothalamus in the brain. Well, as you're sitting there kind of absentmindedly breathing and pressing one nostril at a time, the hypothalamus balances the two nervous systems. When they're balanced, your system runs nice and smoothly, and you want that.

Pranayama is so gentle that it doesn't feel like much as you do it, but as we've just explained, it enriches blood flow to the brain...which is what exercise is all about. You're not cheating when you exercise in this way instead of running around the block 50 times, so don't feel guilty. Detoxification is the point, and pranayama detoxifies you.

Revitalizing Touch: Massage

What with walking a half hour a day, doing some of the yoga positions, and doing a little Vedic breathing, you enrich and purify your body without exerting a lot of effort. Another subtle form of exercise with high-impact benefits is massage. You knead away at knots of stress in your body and feel good doing it.

There is a Vedic form of massage, a technology really, that maximizes the benefits of massage—namely, awakening the intelligence of the body and eliminating impurities. And you can perform it on yourself.

We'll explain a bit more about it in a moment, but first we'd like to address a certain widespread skepticism about whether a little massage is going to do anything at all to prevent something as nasty, mean, and ugly as cancer.

Well, think about it a little bit. Massage involves, first of all, the skin. The skin has pretty much gotten a bum rap until recently in most medical circles. The skin, we all used to think, was just a coating to hold in the body—as if it were armor plating or a plastic bag or something.

The skin is actually an organ, just like the brain, the heart, the spleen, the liver, or, you know, lots of organs that have gotten a lot more favorable ink than the skin until recently. The skin is intelligent. It has all kinds of nerves. One square inch of skin has 78 yards of nerves. Those nerves wouldn't be there unless they were transmitting information, and sending and receiving information involves intelligence. The skin also has pores—20,000 of them in that same square inch of skin that has all the nerves. Pores are for bringing substances into the body (like enriching, rejuvenating oil) and for removing impurities. There are also sweat glands (650 of them in that inch, for coating the skin with water to cool it down), and there are oil glands (one oil gland per hair follicle, with our square inch having 65 hair follicles, on average). Hardly just a coating or cover, the skin is a beehive of activity to benefit the rest of the body.

Skin is one element in massage. The second is oil. You can use a number of different oils in your massage. The massage we recommend for maximum purification—known in Vedic terminology as *abhyanga*—utilizes sesame oil (also coconut oil and olive oil on occasion, but today we'll stick with sesame oil). Sesame oil has a number of health-promoting qualities. First of all, it soaks through the skin really well, so it can work inside the body and not just on the skin. Also, a study by Dr. Edwards Smith found that people who practice daily sesame oil massage have significantly less bacteria on their skin, which may seem like a modest start to preventing cancer. But it's a start. The bacteria killer in sesame oil is probably linoleic acid, which makes up 40 percent of the oil. Linoleic acid is also anti-inflammatory, which is good for keeping your joints working smoothly and helping avert arthritis. The oil as a whole is good for your joints. It lubricates them, which is something that joints really appreciate.

One study has found that sesame oil actually has anti-cancer effects (particularly anti-skin cancer, which makes sense, and also anti-colon cancer effects. The second one doesn't make as much sense right off the bat, but the oil seeps in to reach beyond the surface of the body). Japanese researchers have found that sesame oil contains antioxidants, which, of course, are front line warriors in the fight against cancer.

If you have trouble with standard sesame oil we can recommend a special preparation that should be quite easy on the skin. It's called *Youthful Skin* oil. It's a nice blend of essential oils along with some herbs. Here's what it contains:

Jojoba Oil, Sesame Oil, Almond Oil, Gotu Kola, Sensitive Plant, Silk Cotton Tree, Indian Madder, Woodfordia Floribunda, Indian Asparagus, Albizzia Lebbek, White Museli, Lodh Tree Bark, Indian Barberry, Banyan Tree, Indian Coral Tree, Sacred Lotus, Lemon Oil, Sweet Orange Oil, Coriander Oil, Jasmine Oil.

To find out where to get Youthful Skin oil, see the section at the back of the book called "Product Recommendations."

How does massaging the skin with potent oil purify the body and help fight cancer? You can see right off that the massage would be good for the skin, and it does make your skin soft and lustrous. For purifying the body, just like exercise, oil massage stimulates your body's tissues. When they get active, they refresh themselves. There are channels in the body. Ayurveda calls them shrotas, but Western medicine has nice, familiar names for them—arteries, veins, capillaries, lymphatic channels. The massage loosens impurities, and they then flow out through the channels and the pores conveniently located in the skin. (A warm bath after your oil massage is a good way to open the pores and channels even more and really get the benefit of purification. A warm shower is a second best option. After all, you're going to want to wash the oil off anyway. You can't walk around coated in oil all day. Leave it on for a few minutes if you can, while you shave or cut your nails or something, and then wash it off.) The impurities are also released in the gut for elimination.

If you're going to go sloshing oil all over your body, maybe you'd like to have some method to your madness. Here's the traditional Ayurvedic way to do self-oil massage:

To begin, cure a quantity of sesame oil that you'll use for the next week or two. (Curing makes the oil easier to absorb and increases its antioxidant potency.) Heat the oil in a pan over a low flame. Splash a tiny bit of water into the oil. When you hear the first "pop" of the water, your oil is cured. Let it cool a little, then put the oil into a squeeze bottle to use in your daily abhyangas. (Oh, by the way, don't leave the pan and go off to change the baby or watch the morning news on TV. Wait right by the pan. It will "pop" quickly, and we don't want any random fires from people reading this book.) Here's how to do the actual oil massage:

1. First warm up the oil a little bit. (Warm oil feels better and penetrates better.) Simply place the squeeze bottle in a sink filled with hot tap water for a few minutes. Don't use a microwave. It's fast, but it confuses the molecular structure of the oil.

2. Sit somewhere where you won't cause too big a mess—like in the bathtub or on a piece of oilcloth. Start with your head. Put a little bit of oil in your hands, then—with your hands open and flat—gently rub your head. Mmmmm. Feel that? It's good. Massage in a circular motion. Spend extra time on your head if you like. According to the tradition, massage to the head and the soles of the feet is the most valuable. (In those places there are the most vital points for connecting with the rest of the body and enriching it.)

3. With a little more oil, gently massage your face, also with your hands flat. Go easy on the face. With your fingers, massage your ears. Again, be gentle, but spend some time on the ears. According to the tradition, the ears also influence the whole body. (So they're right up there in importance with the head and the feet.)

4. Massage your neck, front and back, and also the upper part of your back.

5. Massage your arms. (At this point you might think you have a long way to go before you'll do your whole body, but it only takes a few minutes to do the whole procedure.) Use a

straight motion over the long bones but a circular motion over the joints (yes, even the knuckles. You can do it fast.)

6. Massage your chest and stomach. Use a straight motion over the chest and a circular motion over the abdomen. Here, as with your face, don't be too vigorous. Easy is good. Here's a little inside information from ancient tradition—go clockwise over your abdomen. (Your large intestine moves in that same direction.)

7. Rub your lower back and your spine. (Keep getting more oil at each stop.) Here you can be as vigorous as you want. Do your hips, too.

8. Massage your legs the same way you did your arms—straight on the long parts, circular on the joints.

9. Massage your feet. Spend as much time here as you like. As we mentioned, the feet, like the head, connect with all the rest of the body. Close your eyes and enjoy.

You're done. Of course, you're also covered in oil at this point. It's nice to allow the oil to soak in a little if you can. Take a little time to clip your nails, clip your nose hairs, or shave. If you have time, take a warm bath and really let the oil soak in. Or, take a shower. When you're done, let the hot water run a little to flush the oil down the drain.

Oil massage is great in all kinds of ways besides cancer prevention. It's balancing for the physiology, great for the skin, relaxing, fun, and invigorating. Make the oil massage a regular part of your daily routine. At first it might seem messy and annoying, fun as it is. After a few days, though, it can become as welcome a part of your routine as your stewed apple in the morning and your warm milk at night.

A Little Cell "Vacuuming"

Exercise is fine and all that. Even yoga positions are obviously good for you, and, if you close your eyes and listen, you can almost hear them waking up your silent, inner essence. That essence will cleanse itself quite nicely. What if you have some special need, though? Or, what if impurities have built up over

117

a long time, at least a lifetime, and they seem to be a little intransigent. If you begin to think about all the places that impurities can hide in your system, you can start to squirm a little. "Gosh, I'd like to get those out." You can get them in your liver, for starters. They can cruise around your circulatory system. Impurities can be mixed in with your food nutrients, in your muscles, in your fat tissues. Bodily housekeeping can be a big time job.

You can always call for a boost from a food supplement. Licorice is a good purifier. So is Indian Sarsaparilla. But, you don't necessarily do your body a service by having a few licorice sticks and a bottle of the classic old Sarsaparilla pop. For one thing, there's too much sugar in them.

We recommend the supplement named *Elim-Tox-O*. The intent of these tablets isn't just to help move things through the intestines. Lots of internal cleansers do that. Elim-Tox-O, with its specially designed herbs and herbal combinations, targets particular impurities such as:

- Those having to do with the liver and metabolism
- Those having to do with nutrients
- Those related to digestion
- Those related to the eliminative organs

Gee, this supplement even looks to purify your sweat and make it smell better, which you might look upon as a kind of community service. (The "O" in the name refers to "odor.") And it helps produce good, pure blood and fat tissue.

Here's what's in Elim-Tox-O:

Indian Sarsaparilla, Indian Madder (Manjistha), Red Sanders, Siris Tree, Heart-leaved Moonseed (Guduchi), Licorice, East Indian Rosewood, China Root, Ceylon Ironwood, Callicarpa Macrophylla, White Sandalwood, Indian Bedellium (Guggul).

To help give your detoxification plan a boost, take one Elim-Tox-O tablet twice a day for three months. See "Product Recommendations" at the end of the book to find out how to get this.

Facing Elimination

The other technologies we've mentioned already in this chapter do cleanse your system nicely. Walking is great. A few gentle yoga positions are good. The most familiar form of elimination is important as well. You have to have your bowels move regularly. If you don't do that, your impurities sit in the digestive tract, and you reabsorb them. The whole thing is contrary to the idea of detoxification.

A few things help to keep you regular. First, it's good to have the intention to be regular. Begin the day by moving the bowels. You can condition the habit in yourself. Second, eat lots of fresh fruits and vegetables. They will nicely help keep your bowel movements on schedule. The stewed apple to start the day is an excellent fresh fruit, well timed to help keep your bowel movements regular. Third, eat a diet rich in fiber. Finally, exercise helps you be regular in your bowel movements.

Here's a quick summary of what you can do if you have constipation:

- Eat more vegetables
- Eat figs in the morning
- Eat sweet, juicy fruits
- Drink plenty of water
- Use gentle laxative if necessary

"Detox," then, really isn't the clinical process that it sounds like, or something you wouldn't talk about in polite society. Exercise is a big piece of it. Rev up your system a bit, get the oxygen circulating, and let your body detoxify itself. The Vedic tradition teaches exercise that is so gentle that you won't develop shin splints or heat exhaustion, but you *will* rejuvenate yourself.

PART THREE

&

Invisible Invincibility

Nine

Being Nice Is A Spice

Being nice? *Being nice* is going to prevent cancer? Isn't this a stretch by anyone's terms? Well, not by the terms of modern medicine (not that Western medicine goes out of its way to tell you about it as a cancer preventative).

Sixty years ago it was definitely a stretch to think that being virtuous made you healthy. Only physical things caused physical harm, the Western world believed. "Sticks and stones can break my bones," went the knowledge of that time, "but names can never hurt me." Actually, current reasoning goes, names can cause cancer. The interesting insight growing in medical knowledge is that calling *other* people names can make you sick.

Fortunately, modern Western science has begun to establish the connection between negative emotions and disease, and between positive emotions and staying healthy. Most of us have observed that when an elderly spouse dies, often the partner follows shortly after. But for a long time nobody made any connection between the two events, other than saying that "He (or she) died of a broken heart."

Now scientific studies are finding that people who don't feel good mentally also don't feel good physically. People who are depressed have weakened immune systems. They don't have as many killer (NK) cells or other immune cells as happy people.

Gradually, medicine has been accepting this once seemingly farfetched idea that negative emotions are harmful. Know what else is beginning to gain preliminary acceptance? One that everyone finds harder to accept, from medical researchers on down.—The idea that happiness makes you healthier. But that avant-garde idea is also gaining ground. There are strong, increasingly well-documented medical reasons for being happy instead of sad.

Thinking Yourself Sick (Or Well)

Thank goodness for psychoneuroimmunology. Now, since you may be hearing the term for the first time, you may not be quite ready to thank the powers that be for it. But psychoneuroimmunology (PNI) is providing a great service to those who say that being happy makes you healthy and being grumpy makes you sick. The thing is, nobody used to know that smiling had a healthful effect on the body, or that sneering sent ripples of harmful substances through the body.

Now here comes PNI, and it is documenting what its name stands for. "Psycho" refers to the mind, feelings, and moods. "Neuro" refers to your nervous system but also to the neuroendocrine system (which puts out the chemicals that play such a major role in causing or preventing disease). Immunology means the white blood cells and all the various, minute players that keep your body healthy (or unhealthy if they are out of balance). Put the terms altogether, and PNI is the science of formally testing what happens to your body when you hear a good joke, help an old lady across the street, swear, covet your neighbor's snowblower, or have any other kind of thought.

Now, think for a minute about all the advice for right behavior you've ever heard. Ethics have been around forever. Religions have made their recommendations for millennia, and the various religions tend to say the same things, with slight variations. Don't steal. Be nice. Be clean. Be honest.

Before PNI, nobody really thought that the codes of behavior were actually medical advice. Sure, behavior could have consequences in society—if you stole, you might get caught, and you might go to jail. But the popular concept was, "If you steal and don't get caught, you win." Now, PNI is finding that this is not true. Steal, and you create harmful substances in your body, whether you get away with your criminal act or not. On the level of enzymes and neuropeptides, you can't win.

So, what happens in the body when you're mean, rude, hard-hearted, petty, or deceitful in some way? What happens when you do negative things? You shower your body with chemical messengers that can affect your health in a negative way.

First, consider the physical brain and what it does. An area of the brain controls emotions. In popular thinking, we may think of emotions as being in the heart. But science is finding that an area of the brain—the limbic area, which surrounds the hypothalamus—seems to be the actual seat of emotions. The limbic area of the brain controls motivational states, feeding behavior, and those unruly critters (emotions) that sometimes seem to behave as if nothing controls them. Maybe the symbol for Valentine's Day will have to change, to a picture of the limbic area.

The limbic area connects directly with the hypothalamus, and, boy, does that part of the brain do a lot. It's in charge of some physical functions, and that may not be so surprising for a part of the brain that sends out hormones. It takes care of thirst, hunger, blood sugar level, growth, sleeping, and waking. You'd think that would be enough to keep it busy, but it's also in charge of anger and happiness. When somebody cuts you off in traffic and you "go off," the hypothalamus played a part in it, which means that hormones and neuropeptides went coursing all through your body.

The hypothalamus has some potent sidekicks too. It sends out chemical messengers that then get the pituitary gland working (the pituitary is in charge of all your other hormone-producing glands—endocrine glands—for example the thyroid and the most famous of the emotion-related glands, the adrenal glands). The combination of stuff from all these players—hypothalamus, pituitary gland, and other endocrine glands—goes rushing around the body and affects everything. In an instant sometimes. These potent little puppies (the pituitary is about the size of a pea) can make you hot, mad, cold, thirsty, psyched, bored, hostile, in love…and mad combinations of all of them all at the same time.

Fine, the brain and emotions do all these things. But, so what? Surely that couldn't have anything to do with brain cells losing touch with themselves and becoming reckless marauders in your system. Emotions can't cause cancer…can they? Well, here's where the "Immunology" from "Psychoneuroimmunology" comes into play. Neuropeptides from the brain affect digestion (which is why you digest better if you eat in a nice settled atmosphere and aren't watching "Die Hard With a Vengeance" as you eat). They also have complete control over the guys you want on your side when you're fighting disease—the immune system. That's it. That's the connection. Emotions are connected with the army of natural killer cells, interleukins, interferon, all the leukocytes and all of what we scientists refer to as "macrophagic activity." Not only does the brain send messages out to the immune system; the immune system has its own chemicals that carry messages back to the brain. You have a live feedback loop going on in your body at all times, and it responds to the slightest behavior. Gosh, it's almost creepy. It's almost like you're never really alone; your body is always watching.

With respect to cancer, well, immune responses (or the lack of them) mean pretty much everything…the difference between life and death. Here's how to think of the immune system with respect to cancer.—Everybody, it turns out, has some tiny, cancerous cells swimming around at any given moment. It's unnerving to think about, so we won't dwell on it. But it's there. If your body is working up to par, your NK cells dispose of those tiny tumor cells without incident. Smashes them. They're gone, and nobody is the wiser. If the NK cells are too outnumbered, one or more of those tumor cells might continue to grow. And that isn't good. You hate to do anything that might give some of those rogue cells an edge. If your emotions depress your immune system, that gives the bad cells hope.

Depressing Your Immune System

Now, to help make all of this a little more real, take a look at some of the chemicals that our emotions stimulate. One of the more famous chemicals stimulated by the limbic system is cortisol. It regulates your body's response to stress, which is fine as a general principle. However, chronic stress raises cortisol levels, which break down proteins in the body. Know what else it does? "Depresses the immune system," is how we physicians put it. You might not mind the thought of your immune system being a little downcast, but what that phrase really means is that you have fewer lymphocytes, NK cells, and all the cancer fighters. You want some cortisol at the right time, but you don't want it running around like crazy when you don't need it. You won't be able to fight disease as well.

Another big fighter stimulated by the limbic system when your emotions get excited is epinephrine. It's famous. Medicine uses it to combat certain conditions—asthma, for instance. Your adrenal glands are the ones that squirt it out, and it is your "fight or flight" response. You can be standing there, cool as can be, and, wham, you get a shot of epinephrine. Your heart starts pounding. Your muscles gear up. The airways in your lungs open up. It's drastic stuff, and we can all be proud of our bodies for spinning out this substance that completely changes our outlook in the amount of time it takes to have a single thought.

Epinephrine is great. But going around getting all worked up over nothing, and having your body pump out that potent substance, is not going to be the best thing for your physiology in the long run. You should just put out epinephrine when you need it, in the amount you need.

So, you want your cortisol and epinephrine for those times when you are in danger or need some special focus, but you don't want to send them running around all over your body all the time. They'll age you. They'll weaken you. You only want them to appear when you really need them. Otherwise, you overuse them, tire them out, and possibly reduce their power and potential for good.

Favorably Tickling Your Immune System

Well, enough of the doom and gloom. What about the bright side?

Let's start with a joke—how about a short history of medicine, from the medically helpful Website jokes.com.

I have an earache.

2000 B.C.—Here, eat this root.

1000 A.D—That root is heathen, say this prayer.

1850 A.D.— That prayer is superstition, drink this potion.

1940 A.D.—That potion is snake oil, swallow this pill.

1985 A.D— That pill is ineffective, take this antibiotic.

2000 A.D.— That antibiotic is artificial. Here, eat this root.

OK. End of joke. Jokes lighten up your nervous system and send good chemicals floating around. Being happy is a "good drug." When you laugh, your cortisol and epinephrine go down. If you read the first part of the chapter, you know what that means—if your cortisol and epinephrine go down, your NK cells go up. But you don't get healthy just because the bad stuff in your body goes down. Good stuff itself goes up. A good chortle speeds up lymphocyte blastogenesis. (Blastogenesis is reproduction.) In other words, it helps lymph cells reproduce.

We have mentioned that people who grieve a lot tend to die quicker than those who don't. Or, to put this positively, those who handle grief well live longer. Science has validated that, too. According to studies, some upbeat patients with AIDS

128

and cancer outlast those with the downbeat outlook. As some famous old person named W. Osler once put it so nicely, "It is more important to know what sort of patient has the disease, than what sort of disease the patient has."

We recognize some of the seemingly bizarre implications of this analysis. For instance, if you go to the doctor and get told that you have cancer, you should start laughing. Keep on telling jokes. Go on cruises, and enjoy life. Or, if someone close to you dies, laugh a lot at the funeral. Don't dwell on the grief part of it at all, just have a jolly old time. Or, if someone confides in you a particularly sensitive point, such as "My mother is going to die," you immediately start telling jokes. Or how about, you're playing football, and someone gets hit with a shot to the head and goes down. Even as you rush to help the person in all the right medical ways, you laugh and tell jokes. You can picture how unpopular all of this might make you with family, friends, etc., who may interpret it as a lack of respect.

People might think you're insensitive. It is bizarre, and you probably ought to exercise some common sense about it. But there is a learned precedent for fooling around a lot as therapy for being sick. Take Norman Cousins for instance. He was famous. He was editor of the *Saturday Review*, which was also famous. He was diagnosed with a terminal illness ("ankylosing spondylitis," for those who want the hard facts of the matter). He knew a little PNI, though it may not have been called that then. He concluded that his adrenal glands were depressed, so he decided to enliven them. He watched a lot of Marx Brothers movies, which, you have to admit, are pretty funny. And he laughed himself well. He recovered. Although he has passed on now, he nevertheless survived a lot longer than predicted, and laughter did the trick for him.

You don't see a lot of comedy wards in hospitals for people with terminal illnesses, or any other illnesses, for that matter. But maybe you should. "Here's the ER over here." "Here's surgery." "Here's the laughter lab." Good spirits are good for your body.

Charging Up Your "Pharmacological Laboratory"

How do you get your body to make the chemicals that fight cancer and keep it from making the chemicals that give you cancer (and all kinds of other diseases)?

As with many other practical tips we have mentioned in this book, modern medicine is relatively (ok, completely) clueless. "Express emotions," it may say, without knowing quite how to do that so that you maximize the healthy chemicals in your body and minimize the unhealthy ones.

However, Ayurveda specializes in this territory—how to behave so that you create cancer-stopping chemicals and don't create cancer-enriching ones.

Well, basically, ya gotta be nice. It may sound strange. Imagine, for instance, riding a New York subway and smiling at the stranger next to you. This is different behavior, at least in much of our civilization as currently constituted. Imagine going up to a car salesman and saying, "Yes, I put myself in your hands. I trust you." Well, that may be a little extreme. But at least you can be polite to him or her. Being nice is pretty sure to activate your good juices.

"Being nice" is, of course, kind of an oversimplification, though it's a good place to start. Ayurveda has laid out all the rules for the behaviors that increase positive neuropeptides, and here they are:

Behaviors and attitudes to be maximized:
- Love
- Compassion
- Speech that uplifts people
- Cleanliness
- Charity and regular donation
- Religious observance
- Respect towards teachers and elders
- Being positive

- Moderation and self-control, especially with regard to alcohol and sex
- Simplicity

Behaviors and attitudes to be avoided:

- Anger
- Violence
- Harsh or hurtful speech
- Conceit
- Speaking ill of others behind their backs
- Egotism
- Dishonesty
- Coveting another's spouse or wealth

And there it is, in a quick bulleted list—the wisdom of the ages or, as Ayurveda refers to it, *Achar Rasayana*. Now, these items are much easier said than done. What red-blooded world citizen doesn't do a little back biting now and then? (It's hard enough just to be nice to people's faces.) Your cleanliness is bound to slip now and then. (You've been meaning to throw away that old newspaper in the back seat, but you keep putting it off.) You tell a little fib to protect someone's feelings.—Instead of saying, "I don't like you, so I'm not coming," you say, "Gosh, I'd love to come, but I have to clean my goldfish bowl." A little egotism is bound to creep in when your child makes the honor roll and your friend's doesn't. Who can help coveting a little when the neighbor gets a promotion and comes tooling home in a brand new red Jaguar.

Ama and Ojas

It's going to happen. You won't honor these guidelines all the time, but it can be chemically beneficial to move in that direction. In Ayurvedic terms, laughter and positivity don't just decrease cortisol and increase lymphocytes. They decrease ama (the unhealthful substance that clogs your inner channels) and, best of all, they increase ojas—the master coordinator of all activity in your body at even the finest, tiniest levels.

Ojas, in fact, is such a master coordinator that it doesn't just coordinate between, say, one gene and another gene. It doesn't

131

just put the "deoxy" in "deoxyribonucleic acid." It goes a step further. It steps right off into the abyss. Ojas is so smart, so sensitive, so divinely perceptive, it can see the unseen, hear the unheard. It is open to consciousness itself.

The Mistake of the Cell's Intellect

Ayurveda's theory of cancer goes beyond Western theory, which sees cancer as a failure of DNA. Ayurveda sees it as a failure of DNA to reflect the pure intelligence (consciousness) that structures the DNA. In fact, Vedic medicine devotes quite a bit of thought to what it calls *pragyaparadh,* or *mistake of the intellect.* Pragyaparadh refers to the intellect forgetting the memory of its higher Self—the abstract level of consciousness that underlies it, the home of all the laws of nature. The intellect gets lost in the complex, ever-changing vision of the world—the glamour of the material creation—at the expense of the memory of the silent unity of life which is the basis of that creation—the higher Self.

The real risk of cancer comes not just from our intellect forgetting its higher Self, but from each miniscule cell with its miniscule brain (DNA) and its miniscule intellect forgetting the higher Self. Cancer comes about from pragyaparadh of the cell, according to Ayurveda.

How do you get the cell to remember the higher Self? How do you get the cell to have not just healthy DNA but a healthy reflection of the pure consciousness that made it? It would sound like a hard job if you decided to do it. And it is. You have to apply technologies. Those technologies include meditation (which we discuss in the next chapter) and anything that increases ojas, such as laughter.

Here's a tip for the depressed, those who don't like to laugh much, or those who just want to start the day with even more ojas than they'll get from a stewed apple:

"To get rid of depression, walk when the sun is rising." That walk is a very, very powerful way to wake up your cells, to get ojas coursing around, to increase lymphocytes and decrease

132

cortisol. As you're walking, watch the rising sun. (Don't stare at it and blind yourself.) The rising sun is a great event for all of nature. Sun is a lifesaver. Birds rejoice. Trees are thrilled. A welcoming energy fills the air, and it softens the "mistake of the intellect" in your cells. A walk at sunrise might sound pretty simple. But, believe us, it's powerful.

When Nothing But a Pill Will Do

Jokes, right behavior, positive thinking…fine, these things are good. Sometimes a little too much of it can make you gag, but, in general, they are a good cancer preventative. Sometimes, though, all these behavioral approaches seem a bit too indirect and uncertain. Sometimes you want to take a pill, but you would prefer something natural and without side effects.

There is a preparation that you can take to strengthen your immune system if you do find that from time to time your temperament is a little gloomy and you don't always want to be walking around being "little Miss (or Mister) Cheerful." The direct route to some bio-immunity is a tablet called *Bio-Immune,* fittingly enough.

The idea behind these tablets is that you can take certain herbs that directly help the liver work better, purify the blood, increase your resistance to that old troublemaker (stress,) help in assimilating nutrients, and help get your cells talking to each other. (When cells talk to each other, immunity improves. One cell says, "Help." The other understands and comes to its aid.)

In these Bio-Immune tablets there's lots of stuff that fires up the immunity. There's zinc in there. There's mica. There's a little bit of pearl. Here's the complete list of what's in Bio-Immune, for the label readers among us:

Winter Cherry (Ashwagandha), Spreading Hogweed (Punarnava), Picrorrhiza Kurroa, Holy Basil (Tulasi), Centella Asiatica (Gotu-Kola), Embelia Ribes, Neem Leaf, Tinospora Cordifolia Extract, Tinospora Cordifolia Powder, Dry Ginger, Long Pepper (Pippali), Black

Pepper, Mica Bhasma, Mesua Ferrea, Zinc Bhasma, Pearl Bhasma.

Take one to two tablets after breakfast and at bedtime. Continue for three months. See the list "Product Recommendations" at the end of the book to find out how to get it.

A little positivity, then, can pose a serious threat to any cancerous tendencies in your body. A walk at sunrise mobilizes the NK cells, and they briskly go around disposing of tiny little tumor cells. You end up feeling great.

Everybody used to laugh at the idea that being good made you healthy. Well, think of it this way. Science is beginning to show they were not right. Being good does make you strong, and PNI can prove it. But, let's be easy about it. If people's laughing was good-natured and not too jeering, they were increasing NK cells in their body and prolonging life spans. Besides, we have to view them in a good light, or that won't be good for our own levels of cortisol and neuropeptides.

❧ Ten

Meditation Medication

Transcending is a potent cancer fighter...probably *the* most potent cancer fighter, and the one that makes every other cancer fighter work better. But transcending just isn't an everyday thing. Even when most people use the word "transcending," they don't use the same meaning we do here. They mean something like "changing the subject," "ignoring things," or maybe "spacing out for a second" (which is a little closer than the first two choices to what we actually do mean). People look at you quizzically when you mention transcending; or they think they "get it" when, in fact, maybe they get something else.

So we've decided to stick with the widely recognized name "meditation." It would be nice if meditation alone would be all you have to do to prevent cancer. It's a pretty potent cancer preventer all by itself, but in today's world of nasty toxins and bad habits, meditation seems to need assistance from things like diet and spices. Nevertheless, it protects you. In this chapter we explain what transcending is and how it is a kind of launching pad for all kinds of "missiles" in your cancer-prevention arsenal (diet, sleep, etc.). We also explain how transcending makes anti-addiction programs (the ones that haven't helped yet) work very well.

Transcending, Cancer, and You

When you think theoretically about transcending, you can quite readily see it as a powerful antidote for cancerous tendencies in your body. The problem, when it comes to transcending, has been translating the theory into practice—namely, the problem that, since it is rather ephemeral, people think they do it when they don't. We come back to that topic later in this chapter. First, let's talk about what it is. Lots of folks have their favorite literary references to transcending. One of ours is Walt Whitman, who talks of very little else. "If you want me again look for me under your boot-soles," he says. For him to be everywhere (because, presumably, any of us could be stepping anywhere at any moment), he would have to have been an ever-present, universal reality (i.e., the transcendent).

Of course, the transcendent he was experiencing isn't an obvious truth of life to someone who doesn't transcend. For instance, some anonymous wit posted this interpretation of the Whitman line on the Internet: "well, there I was, trudgin' along to class, yu' know, when all of a sudden I felt this *squish,* like I'd just stepped on some little soft-boned, uh, mouse or somethin', so I lifted up my left boot and slowly peeled off this weird, uh—well, sure enough, there he was, a little teeny Walt Whitman, flat as a leaf of grass, only a lot wider."

Walt pictured himself as a *transcendental reality* under the boot soles. Unmanifest. This later interpreter could only picture him as a physical reality, since the interpreter's reality was physical. Laying aside for the moment that transcending is a bit abstract and ephemeral, let's consider briefly the possible anti-cancer implications of transcending.

There is a surface level of the mind where we normally do the things we do when we're awake, such as think about riding the bus, imagine what we'd do if we were in the Bahamas, wish it were the weekend already, solve equations, or guide our hand in steering a car. There's a surface thinking level. For most of humanity most of the time, that's what we know.

Think for a moment about thinking itself, in the same way that physics thinks about matter. Physics sees that matter exists at finer and finer levels. Matter has the structural level, the molecular, the atomic, ...and then the fun really begins. It has subatomic levels, quarks, quanta. A quantum of light is matter yet awfully close to being non-matter at the same time. Now, physics has concluded, beyond the finest level is a unified field of pure, unmanifest energy and intelligence. Physics even offers a mathematical equation—the LaGrangian of the Unified Field—to describe that pure level.

Now, if you're still here, the point is that thinking, like matter, has finer and finer levels and a finest level—pure consciousness. And, one might be tempted to say, the finest level of the mind—the one where Walt Whitman transcends everything—is "like" that unified field from physics. People might be comfortable enough thinking that transcending is "like" the unified field. However, theorists have taken another step and are saying that the field of pure consciousness at the source of thinking, and the unified field described by theoretical physics, are one and the same. They aren't just *like* each other. They *are* each other. And, just as there are laws of nature at the heart of the unified field, as expressed in the LaGrangian, there are laws of nature at the abstract basis of thinking. In fact, *all* laws are in the unified field, and, therefore, *all* laws are at the abstract basis of the mind.

Now here, in theory, is what we're talking about when we allude to transcending—settling the mind into a state where all the laws of nature reside in unmanifest form. That would be worth doing, if you could do it.

The poet Wordsworth (our second favorite English language poet on the transcendent) describes transcending this way:

"...that serene and blessed mood,

"In which the affections gently lead us on,—

"Until, the breath of this corporeal frame

"And even the motion of our human blood

"Almost suspended, we are laid asleep

"In body, and become a living soul:

"While with an eye made quiet by the power

"Of harmony, and the deep power of joy,

"We see into the life of things."

Wordsworth's might be an even better description of transcending than "look for me under your boot soles." But would such a "serene and blessed mood" help fight off cancer? Well, think about it, if you were a living soul with an eye made quiet by the power of harmony, how vulnerable would you be to any disease? The transcendent is the home of all the laws of nature. In other words, it's a field where everything is working right. If you started to get a cold, then you transcended, what chance would the cold have? The cold—or whatever health problem—happens because all the laws of nature aren't working in harmony at one time. Give yourself a good dose of pure laws of nature, and the cold loses its foothold. Just talking about the transcendent doesn't make it a living reality, but it can give us an idea of the possibilities.

Here are some of the ways that transcending would help avert cancer:

- **Transcending and DNA**

   Flawed DNA is the real source of cancer, according to Western medicine. DNA is the brain of the cell; it is the vehicle for directing the cell with intelligence. When you transcend, you soak yourself (and, thereby, your cells) in pure intelligence. This can help correct the flaws in the DNA.

- **Transcending and Phytochemicals**

   Plants have intelligence. Now, we're not being tree huggers here and saying that plants should be protected by equal employment laws. We're not saying that you can talk to them. Plants, like DNA, reflect intelligence. Plants, in fact, have DNA, and plants express their intelligence in protective mechanisms that allow them to survive the harsh effects of intense sunlight, microorganisms, and other challenges. Plants develop their phytochemicals to protect them from their various natural "predators," and you assimilate those phytochemicals when you eat the plants. The chemicals then protect you.

Now, take this another step. The transcendent expresses itself in the plant DNA, and then in the phytochemicals. When you transcend, you take your cells to that most subtle level of creation, where they can fully interact with the most subtle levels of whatever they are digesting. Then, when you have the most intelligence awake within your cells, you are best positioned to derive the most profound level of nutrition from the plants.

- **Transcending and Spices**

   Spices are focused plant intelligence swimming in your body with specific purpose. Their intelligence is looking to awaken the corresponding intelligence in the body. It stands to reason that, the more awake the body's intelligence is already, the better able it will be to enjoy the focused intelligence of the spice. Awakened cells make good spice users, and transcending awakens cells.

- **Transcending and Diet**

   The ideal is to eat whatever you want. Well, if you are reflecting the pure intelligence of the transcendent, you can go ahead and do that. Why? Because what you want to eat will match what you should eat. What you want to eat will be what is absolutely best for every cell of your body. That is, as you soak in pure intelligence, you attune yourself to the laws of nature. Your desires become identical with nature's desires. If you desire a carrot, that's what you need. Such perfect blending of the appetites and what is good for you may be more the experience of the Walt Whitmans or Vedic yogis than of your average world citizen…even the average citizens who transcend. But it's nice to think that meditation nevertheless takes you in the right direction. Also, what we've said of veggies and spices in this chapter is true with diet overall.—Your body naturally assimilates and utilizes all nutrients in the most intelligent way when it has had the advantage of absorbing plenty of transcendental, pure intelligence during regular meditation. And the body is best at ignoring impurities when it is fully awake within itself.

- **Transcending and Sleep**

Everybody knows there's sleep, and then there's real, blissful, energizing *sleep.* If you have trouble sleeping at night, you'll hardly feel as if you're getting the full benefit of an interferon treatment you would get from a good night's sleep. You might have a headache and feel groggy when you wake up in the morning. Your inner pharmaceutical factory won't have been operating at peak levels.

However, if you are in the habit of transcending, and the field of pure intelligence is lively and at work while you sleep, you have a much deeper quality of sleep. You get the interferon that you need. You get the Interleukin-2. You get beneficial neuropeptides that haven't even been discovered yet. You get that sweet nectar that the Vedic tradition describes—ojas. Sleep based in the transcendent is the most powerful sleep there is, and the most powerful cancer fighting sleep.

- **Transcending and the Immune System**

Leukocytes (white blood cells) aren't perfectly smart all by themselves. They just blindly rush around engulfing bacteria, among other things. But you can have too many leukocytes or not enough, and the ones you have may or may not be in peak form. As with the DNA of other cells, get the DNA of the leukocytes reflecting its own inner awareness, and you end up with awesome, unbeatable, perfectly timed, perfectly appropriate leukocytes.

Choose any system of the body, any organ of the body, or any system of the cell, and it will always work its best if it has plenty of the transcendent at its basis; and, it will work worse if it doesn't. Cancer is dumbness at its best (or, if it makes more sense, "at its worst.") It is the lack of intelligence somewhere, compounding itself and becoming lack of intelligence in more places until finally it does what lack of intelligence does...it utterly destroys itself. Consciousness—the transcendent—is pure intelligence. Live it, and your systems thrive. Cancer will find no place to hide.

Transcending...Really, Really Transcending

Transcending—in theory, as we just discussed—is an exceedingly potent experience, well worth having. However, something that calls itself transcending but isn't would hardly be worth the time it took to do it. How do you know what's transcending and what's just ordinary thinking?

Transcending has the misfortune, perhaps, of seeming ephemeral to most people. What's to stop you from saying you're transcending if you're not? The whole thing can cause you to throw your hands up in the air in despair. "What was Whitman doing so that we could find him under our boot soles?" we might ask. "And what can I do so that people can find me under their boot soles?"

Well, as generations of earnest students can attest, you can't have the experience of transcending just by thinking about the experience. Goodness knows, people have tried. They've done their best to convince themselves they were transcending, and they may have convinced some others that they actually were, but they were not.

If you think about Whitman's words but you really have no sense of the transcendent, you picture a fleshy poet squishing beneath your boot sole. Besides, thinking about something means thinking about something. You stay on the surface and think, when what you should do is drop down beneath the surface of the mind to the level where there is no thought. So, thinking about thinking is pretty much a catch-22. It just won't get you to the transcendent, no matter how desperately you want it to do that.

Another candidate for a way to transcend is to "clear the mind of thoughts" or in some other way to focus. Well-meaning spiritual guides offer some such advice often. Most of the popular interpretations of meditation, at least until the last 30 years or so, took "ya gotta concentrate" as their watchword. When the techniques failed, or people just gave up on them because they were boring, the conclusion was, "Well, you just didn't concentrate enough." But when you think about it, concentration is doomed from the outset. When you focus the mind on anything, even on what you may think of as blankness, you focus the mind, right? Focusing tends to hold the mind on a point, when what you want is for the mind to move to the abstract universal (which is no point, you might even say pointless). That is, when you concentrate, you hold the mind on its surface. Yet the whole intent is to go bungee jumping off the surface level of the mind to whatever may lie below. Concentrating won't do it for us, which is quite a relief anyway. Who wants to focus all that hard?

It's popular, as we've mentioned, for people to think that they know how to meditate simply because they are sympathetic to the idea of meditation and close their eyes periodically with the intention of meditating. "It doesn't matter what form of meditation you do," is a popular form of advice these days, even from medical circles. "But at least do something, because it will generate favorable neuropeptides, help your digestion, eliminate impurities, and provide a good basis for combating incipient cancer tendencies in the remote recesses of the body." You hear that a lot, in books that might seem to be much like this one.

But we like to think we're different. Probably any form of closing the eyes and "meditating" does have some good effect, at least compared with the hurly burly of today's busy lifestyle.

Any quietness may be somewhat beneficial in combating cancer tendencies.

However, when you think about what's at stake, it just may matter whether you are genuinely transcending or just closing your eyes and saying you are transcending. You may be able to fool other people but you can't fool the guys that you want to—your own cell nuclei. If you are genuinely transcending, they are bathed in intelligence and feeling heroically energized and enlivened. If you're just sitting there and doing your best to keep your eyes closed, your cells aren't enjoying the same enriching bath with the same potent anti-cancer effect. This shouldn't be any big news flash to anyone. There's real transcending, and there's everything else.

How you meditate matters. It really, really matters. What you really want to do is not simply meditate in some way or another. "How you choose to meditate is really up to you," is often stated and believed these days. No, it's really up to your cells, and they will decide whether you are genuinely meditating or not. They know whether transcending is happening or not, and they respond appropriately, as the situation might dictate.

How do you know if you're really transcending? It may help, in all this, to think in terms of vibration. The universe, as physics is finding, consists of fluctuations of the unified field. It is vibration. It's not just any old vibration, though. For the universe to hold together and continue to work in its infinite complexity, the vibrations have got to be pretty precise. They are, too. They're exact.

The universe starts out as pure consciousness, as we've mentioned. So does your body. Your body *is* pure consciousness. The consciousness resonates within itself, and it resonates in highly precise ways. In the description from physics, the unified field vibrates and becomes photons, quarks and other miniscule particles, then atoms, then molecules, then the dog next door and your front yard and—specific to our conversation—your body.

Think about how vibration manifests in your body. Pure consciousness vibrates in one way, and it's your liver. It vibrates in another way, and it's your pancreas. It vibrates in another way and it's your brain stem...your blood vessels, your stomach lining, your throat,...you get the idea. All that vibrating is extremely precise.

Yes, but do we know what it is? It's Veda (this term means total knowledge for the evolution of life). When pure consciousness vibrates, it produces sound. Ancient *rishis*—or modern ones, for that matter—perceive that vibration and can communicate it. Also, modern rishis can replicate the sounds of the Veda. "Well," you might jest, "can they fix my sore liver by chanting to it?" As a matter of fact, they can, in a technique called "Vedic Vibration."

In one research study on this topic of sound, human cancer cells were grown in the laboratory, and the effect on the cells of a Vedic sound called *Sama Veda* was compared to that of hard rock music. The results showed that Sama Veda decreased the growth of the cancer cells, whereas the hard rock music increased the growth of the cells. Other research gives insight into how sound might have an effect on cells. It indicates that the sound travels through the cell matrix and probably affects the functioning of the DNA of the cells.

Why are we mentioning all this about Veda and vibration and precise sounds? Well, because we would like to give the impression, as physicians, that the technique you use when you meditate matters. You can't just use "any old sound" any more than you would "just throw any old organ into the liver slot." You want a liver where the liver goes, and you want a meditation vibration that truly takes you to that infinitely expanded, caressing, blissful transcendent we've been alluding to.

If your meditation attunes you to your own inner vibration in a precise manner, so that your inner vibration and the universe's vibration resonate with each other in just the right way...that works. You transcend. You become the infinite. People can look for you under their boot soles.

We'd like to call your attention ever so briefly to some scientific research done recently. We're not referring to the entire 6 volumes and 600 studies on Transcendental Meditation as taught by Maharishi Mahesh Yogi. That would be too much to talk about, and hardly anybody would read it anyway. We want to mention just two of the studies on Transcendental Meditation (TM).

Two researchers, Dr. David Orme-Johnson and Dr. Michael Dillbeck, performed what is called a "meta-analysis"—a statistical comparison of 31 scientific studies that measured people doing TM and compared them with people sitting with their eyes closed. What they found was that a whole lot more was going on when people were doing TM than when they were just sitting with their eyes closed. Respiration rate slowed, skin resistance went up, plasma lactate went down (which shows that metabolism has slowed down). The studies haven't had a lot of effect on people saying "it doesn't matter how you meditate, just do it." However, if people did pay attention to scientific studies, they'd conclude from this one that they are better off doing TM than "just any old thing they feel like."

The other study we wanted to mention, published in the *Journal of Clinical Psychology* (by Dr. Kenneth Eppley of Stanford Research Institute International and others) was also a meta-analysis. It tested the widespread idea that various kinds of meditation have as much effect on releasing stress as various other kinds (i.e. "It doesn't matter how you meditate."). Eppley did his meta-analysis on more than 100 studies. He checked out popular favorites like the progressive muscle relaxation technique, and the relaxation response. He found, again, that how you meditate matters. TM reduced anxiety a lot more than any other technique—more than twice as much.

Another study you might like—not a meta-analysis this time—comes from Dr. Nicolai Nicolaevich Lyubimov, Director of the Moscow Brain Research Institute's Laboratory of Neurocybernetics. He found that when people were doing TM, more areas of the cerebral cortex became lively than at other times. For those looking for some physical correlation to transcending, these studies provide great reassurance. During transcending, both hemispheres of the brain become active (according to Dr. Lyubimov). A holistic response happens. An integrated response happens. There are the kinds of expansive effects you would expect if you were transcending...really, really transcending.

How you meditate does matter. The point is actually to "fall asleep" in body and become a living soul. To be there under everybody's boot soles. In short, the point is to transcend. If you do transcend regularly, you are doing the single most powerful thing you can do to fight the possibility that cancer will ever arise in your body. You enliven the one field—the unified field—that enlivens diet, behavior, sleep, and every other form of cancer fighting you might choose to adopt.

Transcending Smoke, Sauce, and Other Nasty Habits

So far we haven't said much about the best-known cancer-causers—tobacco, alcohol, and cigarettes. Here we are, a book on cancer prevention, and we haven't been repeating the litany of "stop smoking, stop smoking, stop smoking." Well, for one thing, the litany just doesn't work. Neither does the litany of "don't drink Seagram's Seven and chase it with a beer." Take any addiction, and the situation is the same. People know it's bad for them, but they just can't help themselves. If they could, it wouldn't be an addiction.

Nobody needs a refresher course on the harmful effects of addiction to the "big three"—cigarettes, alcohol, and drugs. Nevertheless, here is a real quick refresher on tobacco, from the American Cancer Society.—"Smoking is the most preventable cause of death in our society....Tobacco use is responsible for nearly one in five deaths in the United States....Approximately half of all continuing smokers die from diseases caused by smoking. Of these, approximately half die in middle age (35–69), losing an average of 20 to 25 years of life expectancy."

Lung cancer is a particularly revealing "refresher course," because it shows how harmful smoking is and how powerful a little effective prevention would be. Says the American Cancer Society, "Thirty percent of all cancer deaths and 87 percent of lung cancer deaths can be attributed to tobacco." It is estimated that 154,900 people will die of lung cancer this year. For those who smoke, how do the odds stack up? Well, the rate of death from lung cancer is about 22 times higher for men who currently smoke and 12 times higher for women who currently smoke, as compared to those who have never smoked in their lives. (Those aren't great odds.) One of the most encouraging things about lung cancer is that it can be almost totally prevented. One of the most disturbing things about it is that it continues to take so many lives each year.

Meditating, first of all, can actually cut down some of the harmful effects of whatever we might do that builds up toxins in the body. A study by Dr. David Orme-Johnson published in the journal *Psychosomatic Medicine* compared hospital admissions for meditators with those of nonmeditators. Meditators went to the hospital a lot less for almost every disease, including cancer. (As the study put it, admissions were 55.4 percent lower for benign and malignant tumors.)

What about the addictions that cause sickness? Everybody knows that smoking, drinking, and other addictions are harmful. But they feel like doing them. In fact, they feel like doing them so much that they "take just one more, then tomorrow I'll quit."

Society has put together systematic, in-residence programs for overcoming addictions. You go to a facility along with others with the same problem, attend counseling sessions, learn about the multifarious evils of what you have been doing, eventually check out of the clinic, then slip back into the addiction. (Not in every case, of course.) The facilities and programs are in place. We have excellent programs for combating all the addictions. There has been only one problem so far.— They don't work. People enter the facilities because of an uncontrollable urge to smoke, drink, etc. They leave with an arsenal of ways to combat what remains, nevertheless, an uncontrollable urge. The programs are excellent, then, except that they don't root out that deep urge to take something harmful.

Well, what if addicted folks *just didn't feel like smoking* (or drinking, etc.)? What if the pack of cigarettes was sitting right there on the coffee table, the matches were next to it, nobody was around, and the one-time addict just didn't feel like having a cigarette just at that moment? Maybe later. If the urge was gone, then everything else in the current prevention program would really work—the counseling, the literature, the warnings.

Transcending diminishes that urge. Transcending creates that feeling of "I just don't particularly want a cigarette or a drink right now." Think about it for a moment. When you transcend, you bring your mind into contact with an inner field of pure consciousness that is pure "you." You come from there. Your heart cells, liver cells, brain cells, toenail cells come from there. When they transcend, the cells celebrate a little bit. They love it. They feel fulfilled…a least a little bit more than before that moment of transcending. (It doesn't have to be a Whitmanesque, change-the-world-in-a-flash kind of transcending either. Just a little bit of opening the awareness to itself has a big effect.)

When you (and that means your cells) are fulfilled, you don't crave something else. Craving is the uncontrollable seeking after something you don't have. It's a need. When you are a little bit more fulfilled than the moment before, you have a little bit less craving. You are a little bit less…yes…addicted. It is possible, in a natural way, to soften addictions. Transcending fights addiction. It lays the foundation for that anti-addiction program that didn't work before to begin working now.

For the skeptical, who feel that something so slight and ephemeral as a little transcending couldn't counteract something so massive as nicotine addiction, there is quite a lot of research showing that in fact it could. Affirming that TM results in decreased smoking, studies have appeared in *International Journal of the Addictions, Bulletin of the Society of Psychologists in Addictive Behaviors,* and *Alcoholism Treatment Quarterly.*

Perhaps you would have expected the last-mentioned journal to discuss decreased use of alcohol in those who transcend with the TM technique and, in fact, it does. Similar studies showing decreased alcohol addiction in those who practice TM, appear in *American Journal of Psychiatry* and *Journal of Counseling and Development.*

Feeling good already is probably the best way to prevent yourself from reaching for something to make you feel good. Being independent is the best way to keep from being dependent. Transcending makes you feel good. The self opening to the Self is the very definition of independence.

Transcending is a killer cancer fighter. It makes all your other cancer fighting techniques work better—not just a little bit better but way, way better. All the other techniques depend on the intelligence of something—some spice, some rice, some enzyme. Pure intelligence—which you get when you transcend—refreshes, encourages, and enlivens that intelligence of the spice, food, or enzyme. The intelligence of, say, the spice, sees itself in the intelligence of the transcendent, and the two do a little dance together…to the benefit of the cell, and to the extreme detriment of cancerous tendencies. Transcending is good. But to get the benefits of real transcending, you have to participate in real transcending. You don't get points just for nodding your head, saying that you meditate, yet failing to create brain coherence, lower skin resistance, and that serene and blessed mood where you and the infinite have a lot in common.

Eleven

Not Getting Sick from Chemo

"Chemo" therapy is actually "poison" therapy. We don't call it that, because nobody wants to be reminded of what the treatment really is. We use names like "pharmaceutical" or "chemical agent" for the substances administered. The real name, "chemotherapy," is bad enough without using a graphically descriptive name. People dread it. Nobody would willingly go through this therapy except that, when you're sick enough, the alternative is even worse than the treatment.

How do you stay normal, healthy, and vibrant while putting toxins into yourself? Obviously, that's not an easy question. But you can hold your own against chemotherapy.

Everything we've been discussing in this book will help. Everything in this book is natural, so none of it will conflict with your chemo. In this chapter you will find out what chemo is and you will see how some simple, natural things can help keep you stable as you go through the treatment. Diet helps a lot, and a food supplement called *Amrit* has helped quite a few people minimize the side effects of their chemo.

151

Chemo's Bright Side—Pulverizing Cancer Cells

The idea with chemotherapy is to kill or disable cancer cells. Ideally, you would like to kill or disable just your cancer cells. To phrase it politely, chemotherapy interferes with the ability of cancer cells to grow or to multiply themselves. (That is, it poisons the cancer cells.) Because cancer cells tend to be ravenous and selfish, they may gobble up the chemotherapy faster than normal cells. Because the cancer cells are not as well integrated as normal cells, they may get sick and die from the chemo faster than the normal cells. And healthy cells, being basically healthy, are better able than the cancer cells to get back to normal functioning after a chemo assault.

Chemo has a major advantage over surgery and radiation in fighting cancer. Cancer cells can break away from an original tumor and travel to other places in the body. Surgery attacks the original site. So does radiation. Chemo travels in the bloodstream throughout your body. The chemotherapy can locate and destroy the cancer cells wherever they are in the body.

The plus side of chemotherapy, then, is that it makes life miserable for cancer cells. Medicine uses quite a variety of pharmaceuticals for chemotherapy—about 80 of them at the present time—and you may receive a mixture of several. Usually you receive the treatment intravenously (through an IV). You could receive it by mouth or even directly on the skin.

You don't know until you find out from your doctor how long you'll have to be in chemotherapy or how often you'll get the treatments. You may get your therapy daily, weekly, or monthly. Typically, you'll have periods of treatment and periods without treatment, so that your body can rebuild its healthy cells.

But, the point is, yes, chemo can do you some good. Yes, it can even be the only choice. But, gosh, wouldn't it be great if you can poison yourself without, you know, feeling sick?

Chemo's Dark Side—Pulverizing Non-Cancer Cells

Chemo, then, is a great idea from one point of view. The chemo does what you want to do to cancer cells—namely, it kills them. If that were all there were to the story, everyone could just be content with getting chemotherapy whenever necessary. You'd be a little bit uncomfortable with an IV in your arm, but you would treat your cancer.

However, the anti-cancer drugs aren't really selective enough to damage just cancer cells, and that's where the term "side effect" comes into play. The chemicals also damage normal cells. In fact, they can cause quite a bit of damage. In a strange turnabout, anti-cancer chemicals can even torture your normal cells enough to cause cancer in some cases. What kind of cancer treatment is that?

When you think of the chemicals damaging a few cells at the cellular level, the message may not really get through that the substances in your treatment are making you sick. Everyone can afford to have a few cells go bad. But chemo can damage quite a few cells, and the net effect is that not just some cells get sick. *You* get sick. The liver has the job of taking toxins out of your body. Normally it is quite equal to the task. But when you make things miserable for the liver by pumping in toxins through an IV, the liver doesn't stand a chance. It gets overwhelmed. Toxins stay in the body and you feel sick because of them.

Fast-growing healthy cells are the ones most likely to be damaged by chemo. If you're having chemotherapy, you may find yourself with difficulties in your bone marrow, mouth, digestive tract, reproductive organs, even the follicles of your hair. Chemotherapy can mess you up in other places, too—your heart, kidneys, bladder, even your nervous system.

After all, chemo is poison. There are various ways in which chemotherapy kills tumor cells. One popular explanation of how chemo works is that it damages the DNA. In some cases

153

it can increase the number of free radicals in the body—those bandits roaming around in the system that steal electrons from stable atoms and molecules, thereby causing damage to cells. Chemo seems to inundate the cancer cells with free radicals, in the process damaging them. Which is fine, but free radicals are still free radicals. Free is free. These marauders don't know a cancer cell from a healthy one, and they wreak havoc on all fronts.

Sometimes chemotherapy damages your white blood cells, leaving you with a low count of those infection-fighters. A low count of white blood cells means your immune system is weakened. What, then, is going to fight off those routine infections that your healthy immune system disposes of every day? Nothing. During chemo you tend to get infections, most commonly in your mouth, on your skin, and in your lungs, urinary tract, rectum, and reproductive organs.

Not to depress anyone or anything (though depression can be one of the side effects of chemotherapy), but here is a list of some of the common side effects (i.e. sicknesses) that accompany chemo:

- Nausea and vomiting
- Hair loss
- Fatigue (when you need your strength the most, you're losing it)
- Blood problems: anemia, infection, bleeding
- Unpleasant problems with the mouth, gums, and throat
- Diarrhea
- Constipation
- Problems with nerves and muscles (when you're having enough trouble staying calm as it is)
- In your hands and feet, perhaps some tingling or burning sensations, possibly some weakness or numbness there. You may lose balance, feel clumsy, have trouble picking things up or walking, find it hard to button your shirt or blouse, find that your jaw aches, suffer some loss of hearing, and more things.

- You may have trouble with your skin, with such things as itching, redness, peeling, dryness, or acne.
- You may find that, with some drugs, you have bladder irritation or temporary (even permanent) damage to your kidneys. Your urine may change color (orange, red, or yellow) or begin to smell like medicine.

And there's more. You can have...

- Flu symptoms
- Aching muscles, headaches, fever, chills, loss of appetite. (And you don't know if the symptoms are coming from the chemo, an infection or from the cancer.)
- Weight gain (because, instead of losing appetite, you may have cravings)
- Fluid retention
- Puffiness, swelling in your face, hands, feet, or stomach
- Infertility (temporary or permanent)

In general, you may just feel bad all over. In case anyone needed to have it spelled out for them, then, chemo can make a person pretty sick. But, what can you do?

Staying Normal During Chemo: Amrit

There's this stuff called Amrit. It's not a chemical. You don't use it for chemotherapy. You can use it to fight the side effects of chemo. As we've mentioned, chemotherapy poses quite a difficult challenge for the body—to poison bad things but not harm the good ones. Clinical tests have shown that Amrit can help to counter that litany of bad effects from chemo we just listed in the previous section...yet without making the chemo any less effective. That's a tall order, even in our world where prescription drugs can do all kinds of things. Prescription drugs generally can target a single side effect of the chemo and work pretty well on it. Of course, the tradeoff often is that the prescription drug has a side effect of its own. Now, you'll naturally be skeptical about this suggestion at first, but Amrit counters multiple harmful side effects and doesn't introduce any new ones. Clinical tests have shown that to be the case.

The matter of clinical tests is important, for credibility's sake, because Amrit isn't a prescription drug. It isn't even a drug. It's a 100 percent natural combination of ingredients. But its effects have been tested in the laboratory, and the results have appeared in scientific journals.

Humble Cancer Fighter

Amrit, first of all, comes in three forms:
- *Amrit Ambrosia tablets*
- *Amrit Nectar paste* (an herbal fruit concentrate)
- *Amrit Nectar tablets* (a tablet version of the Nectar paste)

To clarify a little bit about these various forms of Amrit, let us begin by explaining that the Amrit Ambrosia and Amrit Nectar do not have the same herbs in them. Consequently, they have different effects on the physiology. With regard to the Amrit Nectar, the Nectar tablets contain all the same herbs as the Nectar paste, but they do not contain several other ingredients that are in the paste, namely, ghee (clarified butter), cane sugar, and honey. The reason for this is that these Nectar tablets were formulated especially for diabetics (who have to carefully monitor their sugar intake) and for patients on chemotherapy (who can have somewhat sensitive stomachs, so the tablet is easier for them to take than the paste).

Now let's talk ingredients. Here's what's in the Amrit Ambrosia tablets:

Meda Milkweed, Black Musale, Heart-leaved Moonseed, East Indian Globe Thistle, Butterfly Pea, Licorice, Vanda Orchid, Elephant Creeper, Indian Wild Pepper.

Here's what's in the Amrit Nectar paste:

Whole Cane Sugar, Indian Gooseberry, Indian Gallnut, Ghee'(Clarified Butter—acts with the whole cane sugar as a carrier to help assimilation), Honey, Cardamom, Cinnamon, Dried Catkins, Indian Pennywort, Cyperus, Nutgrass, White Sandalwood, Aloeweed, Butterfly Pea, Shoe Flower, Licorice, Turmeric. Processed in the aqueous extract of: Castor Root, Country Mallow, Thatch Grass, Eragrostis Cynosuroides, Sugar Cane, Indian Asparagus, Spreading Hogweed, Giant Potato, Winter Cherry, Indian Kudju, Trumpet Flower, Premna Integrifolia, Desmodium Gangeticum, Uraria Picta, Yellow-berried Night Shade, Small Caltrops, Phaseolus Trilobus, Teramnus Labialis, Bengal Quince, Cashmere Bark.

And here's what's in the Amrit Nectar tablets:

The same ingredients as the Amrit Nectar paste, minus the Whole Cane Sugar, the Ghee, and the Honey.

OK, now you're an expert on the various forms of Amrit, right? Well, don't worry if you're not because we are going to tell you a lot more about these powerful formulations. Except for cinnamon and licorice and a couple other ingredients (like cane sugar), these things might seem like just a bunch of exotic weeds to a Westerner. Heart-leaved Moonseed? Not your everyday medicine in America. Thatch grass? Is that good for you? In India, though, these are "hall of fame" type of herbs. Each one is potent.

With Amrit, too, it's not just the ingredients that make the difference. It's the patient, loving, strict preparation. When its makers prepare Amrit, they don't just throw plants into a pot, stew it until it looks right, and then throw it into a bottle. They follow a strict set of steps—no less than 250 steps—that comes from the ancient Vedic tradition. The whole thing is precise and rigorous, even starting with the question of what time of year to harvest an ingredient. (They harvest it only at the time it is most potent.)

OK, forget the Eastern perspective. Think of these pills and paste in Western terms. These modest-looking food supplements are full of phytochemicals (that is, natural chemical ingredients, from plants, that protect against disease):

- Polyphenols (excellent antioxidants)
- Bioflavonoids (natural pigments in fruits and vegetables, known to have many health benefits)

157

- Tannic acid (the stuff in tea)
- Resveratrol (the stuff in wine)
- Catechin
- Alpha-tocopherol (Vitamin E)
- Beta-carotene
- Ascorbate (Vitamin C)
- Riboflavin (Vitamin B_2)

Phytochemicals, though they have no nutritional value, are great cancer fighters. Studies have found that they help slow down cancer-causers (with scary names like nitrosamine) from ever being formed in the first place. When carcinogens do get created, the phytochemicals make it harder for the carcinogens to do their damage. Phytochemicals even slow tumors from growing. These "plant chemicals" ("phyto" just means "plant") are good to have around. Amrit is concentrated phytochemicals.

While we're on this topic, we want to tell you about some of the cancer research that has been done on Amrit. These natural herbs have proved in the laboratory that they can give cancer cells fits and, ultimately, terminate the existence of those troublesome cells.

Studies with mice and rats have shown that Amrit helps prevent cancer, helps reduce tumors when they do exist, and (key for fighting chemo side effects) helps reduce toxicity. Two studies found that the Amrit Nectar paste and the Amrit Ambrosia tablets help prevent and battle experimentally-induced breast cancer in rats. If you're in the mood for some scientific terminology, the studies found that Amrit "protected against...carcinogenesis...by reducing both tumor incidence and multiplicity." Let's go into detail just a little bit more on the study with the Amrit Nectar paste, this time in plain English. The Amrit paste provided 60 percent protection during the initiation phase of the cancer process (this is the phase when the DNA gets irreversibly damaged and the cells become cancerous). Amrit provided up to 88 percent protection during the promotion phase (this is the phase when the cancerous cells grow and increase in number).Another important finding in this study involved the control animals that did not receive the Amrit Nectar paste in their diet.After they developed full tumors, they were then given the Amrit and in 60 percent of these animals the tumors shrank. In half of them the tumor completely disappeared!

Another cancer study looked at the effects of the Amrit Nectar paste on lung cancer in mice.The type of lung cancer researched in this study aggressively metastasizes, that is, it readily spreads. OK, here's the scientific terminology for the results of this study. "The animals receiving [Amrit Nectar paste in their food] had a 65 percent reduction…in the number of metastatic nodules, and a 45 percent reduction…in the size of the nodules, compared to the control group." This means that the Amrit Nectar paste reduced the spread of the lung cancer, and when it did spread, the size of the tumors were smaller.

Liver cancer in mice was also investigated to see if Amrit could provide protection in this area. Some of the mice in this study were fed Amrit Nectar paste and Amrit Ambrosia tablets in their diet, and other mice were not. Liver tumors were produced by giving the mice a chemical called urethane. Results showed that Amrit "inhibits liver carcinogenesis in…mice."To be more specific, there was a 46 percent reduction in the number of mice that developed tumors.

The mice receiving Amrit showed a significant increase in several enzymes that protect the liver functions.The scientific names of these enzymes are glutathione peroxidase, glutathione-S-transferase, and NAD(P)H:quinone reductase.These are good to have around because elevated levels of these enzymes are linked with preventing mutations caused by carcinogens.They are also linked with blocking toxic effects and tumor-producing capabilities of carcinogens.

Another interesting finding in this study was a significant increase in the expression of gap junctions between cells, in the mice that ate Amrit. These gap junctions are specialized membrane channels made of integral membrane proteins called connexins. Connexins are important because they help cells communicate with each other. During carcinogenesis this communication process is hindered. By increasing the number of connexins, communication improves between the cells and this helps to prevent tumor formation.

Preventing cancer or stopping it from getting worse is imaginable. Turning cancer cells back into normal cells sounds pretty impossible. In fact, medicine has held it as a truism that you just can't do that. Once the DNA gets damaged, forget about it. It's a Humpty Dumpty kind of thing. Or is it? Studies done on cancer cells grown in the laboratory found that Amrit caused cells headed in the cancerous direction to change their minds, so to speak. Amazingly, there was a "reversal of the malignant process."

One of these studies investigated a type of nervous system cancer called neuroblastoma. Normal nerve cells are long, with round central bodies and long projections. When they become cancerous, their central bodies shrink and they lose their characteristic projections. As a result, they appear round instead of long. In this experiment, extracts of the Amrit Ambrosia tablets were added to the mouse neuroblastoma cells and, voilà, the cells became long again. They formed projections once again. They also started to function chemically the way normal cells do, producing enzymes they had stopped producing.

It's rather like taking criminals and restoring their brains so they don't think like criminals anymore but like nice, socially well-adjusted people. This synergistic combination of herbs actually turned bad nerve cells back into good ones.

A similar study was done on another type of cancer called melanoma, which occurs in cells that produce the pigment called melanin (this pigment is commonly found in your skin and eyes). These melanin-producing cells look similar to nerve cells, with the round bodies and the long projections. When they become cancerous, the same thing happens to them that

160

happens to the nerve cells — the round bodies shrink and the cells lose their much-needed projections. In this study, when extracts of Amrit Ambrosia tablets were added to the melanoma cells, their round bodies got larger and they formed the long projections again. They came back to normal. The growth of the melanoma cells was also inhibited by extracts of Amrit Ambrosia tablets and Amrit Nectar paste.

Immunity Booster

A sound immune system is essential for good health and prevention of cancer. Several studies done on Amrit show that it boosts immunity. Amrit Ambrosia tablets and Amrit Nectar paste both improve the responsiveness of lymphocytes and macrophages (these are two types of immune system cells). By "responsiveness" we mean, How well do these guys respond when a challenge is put to them? Well, under laboratory conditions, the increase in lymphocyte responsiveness was as much as 3–4 times higher in mice that were fed Amrit. Also, there was a significantly increased production of Interleukin-2 by lymphocytes from mice fed Amrit Nectar paste.

When macrophages (which gobble up any number of things, including bacteria and cancer cells) from mice that were fed Amrit Ambrosia tablets were activated by different biochemicals, they had a much greater ability to destroy tumor cells. In addition, the production of nitric oxide in these activated macrophages was much higher. This is an important finding since nitric oxide is considered a key player in the process used by macrophages to destroy bacteria and tumor cells.

Battling Chemo's Side Effects

This stuff battles cancer in mice and rats, which attracts our attention. It strengthens immunity, which has got to be a good thing. This combination of exotic, funny-sounding herbs seems healthy. How is Amrit in fighting the battle we're concerned with in this chapter—chemotherapy toxicity? Pretty good, it turns out....Some studies, for instance, have looked at how well

Amrit can help dispel the side effects of particular drugs used in chemo. Cisplatin, for one, is good for testicular, ovarian, and other cancers. But, being poison and all, it does have toxic side effects. A study of the Amrit Nectar paste showed that the nifty blend of Indian herbs works to reverse those effects.

Here's what happens when Cisplatin is given. It tends to decrease glutathione (GSH) and glutathione-S-transferase (GST) activity in both the liver and the kidneys. And those are two chemicals that your body doesn't want to be without. Glutathione has the heady responsibility of protecting your liver function. It helps the liver remove toxins such as alcohol, drugs, pollutants, and other poisons. Glutathione also protects the liver from getting cancer. As if all that wasn't enough, glutathione is needed to keep your immune system healthy. Laboratory studies have shown that it stimulates the production of both Interleukin-1 and Interleukin-2.

We've already talked a great deal about Interleukin-2 in this book, so you probably know that it's involved in helping immune cells grow and multiply. Interleukin-1 is an important player in the immunity game as well. It's involved in the inflammatory response that is necessary for fighting infections. What about glutathione-S-transferase? Why is it so important? Well, it is also involved in ridding your body of toxins, and, even more relevant to this book's topic, it protects healthy cells from getting cancer.

OK, back to the Cisplatin study. The results showed that Cisplatin did not decrease GSH and GST levels in the livers and kidneys of rats that were fed Amrit Nectar paste in their diet. Amrit maintained healthy levels of glutathione and glutathione-S-transferase in both the liver and the kidneys. That's a result the body certainly welcomes.

Another chemotherapy drug, Adriamycin, can damage the heart, even causing death. Adriamycin damages the DNA in cancer cells, which is good. However, it produces tons of free radicals that damage the heart (which, of course, isn't good). In a study on mice, 60 percent of the mice that didn't take

Amrit Nectar paste died from Adriamycin, while only 20 percent of the ones that did take the Amrit died—a significant improvement in the survival rate.

What about the question at hand here? Does Amrit help the side effects of chemo in patients? Again, there have been studies, since nobody believes anything unless there have been systematic measurements, and experiments using controls and all that.

One study was conducted on 62 patients with different types of cancer who were undergoing intensive chemotherapy. One group of patients took Amrit Ambrosia tablets and Amrit Nectar paste along with their chemotherapy, while the other group did not. The patients who took Amrit got relief from several different side effects. Amrit reduced vomiting, reduced diarrhea, and reduced blood toxicity (chemo can sometimes be lethal to some of your blood cells). Any relief is good. These findings alone seem worth the price of admission. But, wait, there's more. Amrit also improved sleep (a great anti-cancer tool in itself), improved body weight, and helped improve the patients' overall sense of well-being.

Another study was conducted on 129 breast cancer patients who were undergoing chemotherapy. These patients were randomly assigned to one of two groups. There was a group who took Amrit Ambrosia tablets and Amrit Nectar paste, and there was a control group who did not take Amrit. Once again, this study found that Amrit reduced side effects of the chemotherapy. The patients who took Amrit experienced:

- Decreased anorexia (loss of appetite)
- Decreased vomiting
- Improved scores on the Karnofsky Performance scale (not that anybody cares about the name, but this test measures the ability to perform normal daily activities, and everybody cares about that.)
- Improved general well-being

163

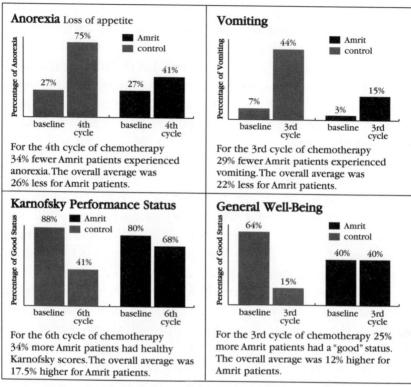

Bar graphs reprinted with permission from Townsend Letter for Doctors and Patients, *August/September 2000, pp. 134–138, Tel. 360-385-6021.*

But how could Amrit resolve the paralyzing catch-22 it encounters? Chemo, of course, is supposed to make cancer cells sick. Amrit makes you healthy. How does it let the chemo do its necessary, if distasteful, work while making you feel better in spite of the poisons you've introduced?

Somehow it does. In the study on breast cancer patients, tumors shrank just as much in the Amrit group as the non-Amrit group. The chemotherapy still worked.

There's currently a lively controversy brewing in the medical community over this very issue. There's a belief among some oncologists (doctors who treat cancer) that taking antioxidants such as Vitamin C, Vitamin E, and beta-carotene will prevent the anti-tumor effect of chemotherapy by neutralizing free radicals. Research has not yet provided a definitive resolution to this controversy when it comes to the use of isolated synthetic antioxidants (this is a fancy scientific term for the tablets of Vitamin C, Vitamin E, beta-carotene, etc. that you buy at the store), but this argument doesn't hold any weight when it comes to Amrit. Research has proven that.

To widen the scope of this discussion a little bit, we would like you to know that it is better, in general, to use natural forms of antioxidants (such as those in foods or herbs) instead of the synthetic type. The body can assimilate the natural forms much better. And, according to Ayurveda, combinations of natural antioxidants (such as those found in the Ayurvedic herbal mixtures) are much more beneficial than single isolated antioxidants. The various herbs in the Ayurvedic mixtures work together in a synergistic manner to yield a powerful effect. At the same time, there are herbs in these mixtures that prevent any adverse side effects from occurring.

Synthetic, isolated antioxidants can sometimes have unexpected adverse effects. For example, there are conflicting reports in the scientific journals regarding the usefulness of beta-carotene in preventing lung cancer. Some studies indicate that beta-carotene is helpful in preventing cancer, while some research indicates it may actually worsen the scenario. However, the scientific evidence is clear-cut when it comes to the matter of getting your antioxidants from food. The incidence of cancer is definitely lower in people who eat predominantly vegetables and fruits in their diet.

As we're sure you know by now, vegetables and fruits contain lots of phytochemicals, such as polyphenols and bioflavonoids—the plant-based chemicals that have antioxidant and DNA-protective qualities, as well as a large number of other beneficial activities. Herbs take it up a notch to the next level. They contain even higher concentrations of these wonderful phytochemicals. The proper combination of herbs—like the combination found in Amrit—yields a concentrated mixture of phytochemicals that produces anti-cancer effects and protects against chemotherapy toxicity. And Amrit does all this without compromising the anti-tumor effect of the chemotherapy.

One theory on how Amrit pulls this off without a hitch, involves a basic difference between cancer cells and normal cells. The cell membrane (the "skin" of the cell) is composed of saturated fatty acids in most cancer cells, while normal cell membranes are made of a different type called polyunsaturated fatty acids. Saturated fatty acids cannot be oxidized by free radicals. Therefore, the cancer cells are not protected by antioxidants, and the anti-tumor effects of the chemotherapy continue without hindrance. Normal cell membranes (containing the polyunsaturated fatty acids) can be oxidized and this damage results in the toxic side effects of chemotherapy. Antioxidants can prevent this damage to the normal cells by stopping the oxidation. So, the antioxidants found in Amrit not only protect and defend the normal cells, but also allow the chemotherapy to continue its battle with the cancer cells.

Don't forget, Amrit also maintains healthy levels of glutathione and glutathione-S-transferase in the physiology. As we discussed before, these chemicals help remove toxins from the body, thus reducing the toxicity of chemotherapy. Also, Amrit is composed of a mixture of phytochemicals and all the functions of these plant-based chemicals are not yet known. There may be other mechanisms by which Amrit provides protection against chemotherapy.

Amrit—How to Take It

How much Amrit should a chemotherapy patient take? Twice as much as the normal recommended dosage. Here's what to take:

- 1 Tablespoonful (20 grams) of the Amrit Nectar paste twice a day **or** 2 Amrit Nectar tablets twice a day
- 2 Amrit Ambrosia tablets twice a day

More Ways to Stay Normal

Everything in this book is about keeping yourself balanced, normal, and healthy. Everything in here will help you keep from getting sick during chemotherapy. Here are some more things that you can do so you don't get depressed, nauseous, and otherwise out of sorts while you're doing what you have to do to battle cancer.

- **Transcendental Meditation**

  Meditation gets you rested, battles stress, bathes your cells in intelligence, helps you focus, and in many other ways keeps you grounded and alert as you fight the battle of your life. A large percentage of chemo patients—as many as half—start to feel a little nauseous even before they start treatment. Well, clearly, that's mental. Mental techniques such as meditation are a great way to counteract mental problems.

- **Sesame Oil Massage**

  You don't want errant free radicals even as your chemo creates free radicals to fight the cancer. Sesame oil massage works through that elaborate organ of the body—the skin—to bring reinforcements to your body's fight to maintain its equilibrium. Do sesame oil massage at least once a day, and take a warm bath while the oil is on your skin. The bath opens the pores and lets the rejuvenating oil seep in. One cautionary note, though—don't do the oil massage if your white blood cell count is low.

- **Veggie Diet**

  Bombard yourself with phytochemicals. Phytochemicals help the plants resist poisons. You want to resist the wrong toxins in your body, even as your chemotherapy goes to work on the sick cells in your body. You want to strengthen the healthy cells so they can recover quickly from chemo.

  Enjoy broccoli and its brothers (cauliflower, cabbage, Brussels sprouts, kohlrabi). These folks have chemicals called indoles, which make estrogen less effective (seeming to reduce the risk of breast cancer).They also seem to stimulate the body to make anti-cancer enzymes.

Allow yourself some allium vegetables (garlic, onions, leeks, and chives).They have allyl sulfides in them, and the suspicion in scientific circles is that these sulfides block chemicals that cause cancer.You want them working side by side with your chemo as you fight the cells that have gone wild.

Seek out some citrus. Limonene in these fruits sparks enzymes that, we suspect, help the body get rid of carcinogens.

Grab some grains.These have phytic acid, which binds to iron; that action, we suspect, may help cut down on excess free radicals.

Fill up on fruits. Caffeic acid in fruits helps produce an enzyme that assists your body in flushing out carcinogens. Ferulic acid has a fine effect chemically. It binds to nitrates, perhaps keeping those chemicals from turning into cancer-causing nitrosamines.

During chemotherapy you want your prescribed chemicals to work according to plan. Other than that, you want to be as normal as you can possibly be. Food won't interfere with your chemo, and it will help keep you normal. So, go for all the fiber, beta-carotene, Vitamin C, folic acid, and allyl sulfide you can get.Value your vegetables.

- **Exercise**

   Like you feel like exercising when you have those helpful toxins in your body, right? Exercise is the great purifier. Just walking a half hour a day is all you need.You may find yourself feeling better about yourself as you move about.Walk at sunrise if that works out for you, and you'll find yourself cheering up. (The walk at sunrise is an ancient Vedic technique to combat depression.)

   Some of the Vedic forms of exercise, presented in Chapter 8, don't really involve any effort to speak of.And they can smooth you out and revitalize you.Try a few gentle yoga asanas to get your mind and body working in unison. Do the breathing technique called pranayama. It revives the brain and refreshes you overall, and all you do is close your eyes, move your fingers a little bit, and breathe (as explained in Chapter 8).

- **Turmeric**

    Simple-looking little turmeric is potent stuff. It protects your DNA. It stimulates an enzyme (glutathione S-transferase) that gets rid of toxins and protects healthy cells against cancer. It helps keep down inflammation. It helps your phytonutrients be even better at fighting cancer than they are naturally. It fights bacteria. It is just, flat out, a good way to address all kinds of side effects of chemotherapy.

- **Sleep**

    Your body is a chemical factory that knows more than your doctor, more than anybody about keeping itself balanced, normal, and healthy. When you're awake, the chemical factory has so many processes going on that it gets fairly overwhelmed. When you're asleep, the chemical factory focuses strictly on restoring and revitalizing you. Max out your beneficial neuropeptides by getting a full night's sleep.

An Rx to Keep You Well During Chemo

It's nice to combine all the advice from this chapter into a simple list you can follow each day as you go through your treatment, with a couple fresh points besides. Here is a simple regimen to help keep you well as you undergo chemotherapy:

1. Drink lemon and honey water in the morning. (It's purifying. Lemon, we mentioned earlier, has limonene.) In one glass of water have about 1 tsp. lemon juice and 1–2 tsp. honey.
2. Eat turmeric. Have 1 tsp. of turmeric sautéed in ghee (clarified butter) or olive oil, three times a day.

169

3. Follow these diet recommendations:
   - Eat veggies: Lots of squash, cauliflower, cabbage, cucumber, basil, zucchini, asparagus, green beans, plantain, spinach, artichoke, green papaya, green leafy vegetables.
   - Enjoy lots of sweet, juicy fruits.
   - Take moong dal—it's full of protein and easy to digest.
   - Have lots of grains—whole grains, barley, couscous.
   - Avoid these things: Hot and spicy foods, vinegar, excess salt, sour foods, fermented foods, and deep-fried foods. These foods stimulate the digestive enzymes in your body at a time that you want to quiet such enzymes and maintain balance in your physiology.
4. Take Amrit (rich in phytochemicals).
5. Meditate twice a day.
6. Massage with sesame oil once a day, usually in the morning.
7. Enjoy a nice walk for half an hour each day, at sunrise if possible.
8. Get a good night's sleep.

Sometimes in life we just have to "bite the bullet"—hunker down and do something distasteful so that we benefit in the long run. Chemotherapy is such a thing. It is definitely distasteful but, when you have cancer and it has spread, then chemo beats the alternative of staying sick. In the past, the side effects have been perhaps the worst part about chemotherapy.—If your own sickness didn't get you down, the treatment probably would.

But a few simple things are surprisingly powerful in helping keep you healthy and sane as the chemicals help your body get rid of cancer. Good diet. Exercise. Meditation. Amrit. These are small, gentle things to add to your routine. But these simple things really have a big effect. The prospect of chemo is not nearly so daunting when you know you can go through it without necessarily getting so sick.

❦ Twelve

The Answer to Anything

I f our cancer-fighting recommendations were just for fighting cancer, who would bother with them? "Hey, I don't have cancer today," we happily think, "and, if I do, I don't know about it." You just don't go around preparing yourself against the 50 percent chance of cancer that might happen 30 or 50 or 100 years down the road. And speaking of "road," we generally figure we'll probably get hit by a car long before we ever get cancer.

So, if the recommendations in this treatise were simply to prevent that long-term, often-deadly, virulent disease nobody even likes to *think* about…well, then, fuhgeddabouddit. Who would do these things? We just don't particularly walk around preventing cancer any more than we go out of our way to avoid falling boulders on the highway, random arrows from archery ranges, foul balls from nearby baseball parks, or runaway trains coming through our front yards. Most calamities are remote and besides, we don't want to think about them. It's unpleasant, and that increases cortisol. (See Chapter 9, "Being Nice is a Spice.")

Cancer prevention isn't just *cancer* prevention. It is, pure and simple, prevention. It's *everything* prevention. The techniques and procedures in this book enrich health...all health.

Think about it this way. Cancer is the disease that comes from the deepest level of your body. It's a disease of the DNA. Heart disease, which nobody wants to get, is generally a disease of the blood vessels (not from as deep a level as cancer). Arthritis is a disease of the joints, though coming from some deeper imbalance. A cold is, among other things, a sickness of the nose (or, more technically, the sinuses). A stomachache may be a problem from a chemical imbalance inside you.

Cancer—scary, unsolvable cancer—is a sickness from the deepest level. It is a mix-up in the DNA, that chemical brain center of the cell and, thereby, of your body. It is very, very difficult to adjust the body at the level of the DNA, which is why Western medicine, for the most part, just doesn't try when it deals with cancer. It performs surgery, radiation, and chemotherapy at the structural level of the body and then sends the cancer patient on his or her way.

However, the prescriptions in this book challenge cancer at that deepest level—the level of the DNA and the source of the DNA, the body's own intelligence. And here is the logic we are following. If you fix imbalances at the deepest level, you fix them at all the ensuing levels as well. If your DNA is healthy, and your DNA is everywhere in your body, then your digestion is healthy, your brain is healthy, your heart is healthy, your skin is healthy, your big toe is healthy (and the toenail right along with it). *You* are healthy.

Let's look at the same discussion in terms of that modern pest now being blamed for so many problems in the body— free radicals. Free radicals seem to cause cancer, as we've mentioned. They seem to cause heart disease, by damaging blood vessels. They contribute to infections, because they weaken the immune system's ability to fight infections. If they weaken the immune system, then they contribute to all kinds of diseases that arise when the immune system can't get its job done. The simple procedures in this book, chapter after chapter, dramatically decrease free radicals in the body, and that means that they cut down sickness in general (not just sickness from cancer). Phytochemicals (from the vegetarian diet) are a systematic assault on free radicals. Sleep challenges and disposes of free radicals. Amrit has a lab-proven ability to decimate free radicals (without interfering with chemotherapy). So, if you view sickness from the perspective of free radicals, the suggestions in this book would seem to help fight all disease.

Let's just look at some of the specific ways you are taking care of your overall health when you are taking on preventative, cancer-fighting measures.

Dismissing Heart Disease

Heart disease is still the number one killer in America and elsewhere, though the world is making progress against it. Much of what gets done is reminiscent of the approaches to cancer—namely, surgery. (Does the term "bypass" suggest anything?)

However, heart disease is every bit as preventable as cancer. And—here is the point—the techniques in this book to prevent cancer also, unconsciously, help to rule out heart disease. Think about some of the approaches from this book and what they might mean against heart disease:

- **Diet**

    Fatty diet, we have come to understand, is the culprit in much of heart disease. Blood vessels become clogged, blood no longer flows as well through those constricted vessels, the heart has to overwork itself, and disaster ensues. The diet recommendations in this book are totally healthy for the heart. You don't have to eat one diet to prevent cancer and another to prevent heart disease. The stewed apple you eat to start the day, rich in soluble fiber, helps to lower cholesterol. Vegetables, rich in indoles and folate, are low in fat. Whole grains are regular "roto rooters" against cholesterol. The "don't die yet" diet wouldn't have much value if it kept you from dying from cancer but let you die from heart disease, would it? Well, it does have value.

- **Exercise**

  Exercise is another staple of the "anti-heart disease" community. Occasionally joggers drop dead while running, and more than one person has been launched into a crisis while walking the treadmill in a doctor's stress test. Modern medicine may not have a good handle on the gentler forms of exercise. Nevertheless, if properly done, exercise strengthens the heart and unclogs the blood vessels. Well, this book is strong in recommendations for gentle, careful exercise that enriches the cells without strain—walking, yoga positions, morning massage. Great against cancer, these techniques are superb against heart disease as well.

- **Meditation**

  Stress, the world has belatedly come to recognize, causes illnesses like heart attacks and stroke. Before, thinking there was no antidote to stress, we all just plunged on ahead and let the stuff accumulate in our lives (especially in our hearts). About the only escape from stress was a heart attack, which was only a temporary relief at best (and often proved fatal). Now we have systematic rest as an antidote to stress, and studies have shown that the rest during Transcendental Meditation is deeper than that in the deepest sleep.

  Scientific studies have found, repeatedly, that meditation helps lower blood pressure—another great heart attack preventative. Meditation is a holistic form of rest and rejuvenation that, being good for you overall, is good for your heart.

- **Spices**

  Turmeric, of which we've made a great deal in Chapter 4, is good for your digestion, which means that it will help to dissolve undesirable fats in your body instead of allowing them to accumulate. This yellow spice is a supremo antioxidant. It gobbles up free radicals, which in turn protects your blood vessels. It's antibacterial, and it's always good for the heart to cut down on the infection-causing bacteria in the system. Do you think it's good for your heart to eat turmeric regularly as a cancer-preventative? Well, it is.

- **Sleep**

Given the chance, your body's chemical factory really goes to work to counteract problems while maximizing benefits. Sleep gives the body that chance. Just as there are neuropeptides that are key in the fight against cancer, there are neuropeptides that strengthen the heart and the blood vessels. During sleep the body can get down to the valuable task of producing them…without a lot of interference from your overactive mind.

- **Being Nice**

Speaking of neuropeptides, being nice is a great way to send beneficial chemicals coursing through your arteries. People often speak of emotional problems as giving pain to the heart, and such description is not just a quaint metaphor from the past. Anger and mean behavior is bad for the heart. Love, compassion, and nice behavior is good for the heart.

- **Amrit**

Free radicals have a field day damaging your blood vessels, and that isn't good. Amrit, which gobbles free radicals, is an across-the-board protection against heart disease. There have been research studies done on various aspects of heart disease to see what effect Amrit has in this area. As with the cancer research, the results have been astounding.

A clinical study was done on patients who have high levels of cholesterol in their blood. The patients who took Amrit Nectar paste and Amrit Ambrosia tablets got positive results. They had a much higher resistance to oxidation of their low-density lipoprotein (LDL—the bad type of cholesterol). In other words, Amrit protected the LDL from getting oxidized, or damaged, by free radicals. This is definitely beneficial because once the LDL gets oxidized, it becomes toxic and contributes to the process of atherosclerosis (this is a fancy name for hardening of the blood vessels) in which plaques form along the blood vessel walls and obstruct the flow of blood. Protecting the LDL from oxidation is a crucial step in preventing heart disease. As compared to Vitamin C, Vitamin E, and a drug, Amrit has been found to be at least 1000 times more potent as a free radical scavenger in protecting LDL from oxidation.

You hear so much about cholesterol these days— good cholesterol, bad cholesterol, high cholesterol, low cholesterol. Understand this—cholesterol, in and of itself, is not bad. Matter of fact, you need cholesterol for a lot of different functions in your body. Know where the highest concentration of cholesterol in your body is? Your brain. Yes, your noggin needs cholesterol. And if your cholesterol level gets too low, your brain may feel the effects. So you don't want cholesterol levels that are too low.

You also don't want cholesterol levels that are too high. The reason for this is that high levels of cholesterol give rise to higher concentrations of oxidized cholesterol, which is toxic and damages the blood vessels. An everyday way of understanding this is to consider your car. You get the oil changed every 3–5 thousand miles, right? Well, even if you don't, you're supposed to. Why is it important to change the oil at regular intervals? Because the oil in your car gets oxidized and can eventually clog and damage the engine. Similarly, the oil in your body (cholesterol) can get oxidized and damage your blood vessels. Amrit stops this process.

Let's talk about another study done on Amrit. This one was done on Watanabe rabbits, a special type of rabbits that normally have very high cholesterol levels and consequently get atheroma early in their life. Atheroma is scientific lingo for the plaques we mentioned above. These plaques can eventually result in complete blockage of the blood vessels, and then a heart attack can occur. Amrit Nectar paste reduced the formation of these plaques in the Watanabe rabbits that ate Amrit in their diet. In spite of extremely high cholesterol levels, Amrit reduced the formation of atheroma by as much as 53 percent in these rabbits. This finding correlates well with the results of the study we talked about above. Amrit protects the cholesterol from getting oxidized, therefore preventing plaques in the blood vessels from being formed.

Another symptom of heart disease is called angina. Patients with angina get pain in their chest when they overexert themselves. A clinical study was done on these patients and the ones who took Amrit Nectar paste and Amrit Ambrosia tablets had fewer episodes of angina. And when they did get angina, the pain was less severe.

"Why don't you just say that every technique in this book is as good for the heart as it is for cancer prevention?" you might reasonably ask at this point. We would say that you have an excellent point. Every technique in this book is an anti-heart disease technique as well as an anti-cancer technique. We can't think of a single exception to this rule. Fighting cancer means fighting heart disease. It's a great two-pronged assault on deadly killers.

Disposing of Bad Digestion

A whole category of illnesses has to do with eating. We can't get enough of foods, it seems, especially the wrong ones— processed foods, fatty foods, sugar. The gentle procedures in this book combat the recurring, annoying, un-cosmetic disorders that have to do with eating. Here is some of how that works:

- That stewed apple first thing, as the sun peeks over the horizon, sets the digestion for the whole day. Small apple, big benefit. Your digestion begins to take the right angle even before your first cup of coffee (which you shouldn't be having anymore) or your bacon and eggs (also not particularly healthy for you).
- Turmeric assists digestion and fights harmful bacteria (which can wreak havoc in your mouth, stomach, and other parts of the digestive tract).
- Breaking the sugar addiction is really powerful in fighting obesity, or even that extra inch around the middle or the unwanted fold under the chin. It is also a good way to minimize the likelihood that diabetes will rear its ugly head.
- Veggie diet, or at least a diet with less meat than before, eases digestion…especially if you cook the vegetables to ease the burden on your digestive enzymes. And the veggie diet cuts down on animal fat, which helps cut down on the fat stored in your own body.
- The morning apple, as well as the rich fiber in your vegetables and grains, has the added side effect of tending to eliminate constipation—another chronic problem for much of the general population.
- Herbal Digest, the modest little food supplement we spoke of in Chapter 5. Sometimes, even though you're doing everything right, your digestion doesn't get it done quite the way it should. It's not cheating to mix into the diet a preparation of natural ingredients. After all, pomegranate seeds are still natural, even if you happen to take them in an Herbal Digest pill. So, for those with reluctant stomachs in one form or another, a little Herbal Digest can prod the system in the direction of lightness, vitality, and balance (all good things when you're talking about digestion).

Digestion is pretty central to how you feel. Get it working right, and you're on top of the world. Well, do the things in this book, and you'll get it working right. Stop eating the burger and shake every noon. Eat some delicious cooked veggies instead, and you won't be arguing with your stomach all afternoon.

Conquering Colds

Colds, flu, and infections are kind of a catch-all form of disease. Aside from the fact that everybody seems to catch them, they seem to occur without any real explanation or any real cure.

Often, a cold or any of its sister ailments is actually the expression that too many impurities have built up in the body. Ayurveda is fond of saying that ama has built up. Everything in this book conspires against that annoying, destructive accumulation of impurities in the body. Such impurities over the long term can become the worst health fate of all—cancer. Such impurities over the short term can mean...a cold. Or, to put this into a positive light, eliminating impurities means eliminating that other most unsolvable of all ailments (besides cancer)—namely, the common cold.

Here is how a few of the practices in this book help to fight colds and flu:

- **Sleep**

    Your mom knew what she was talking about. Get proper rest, and you don't get sick.

- **Diet**

    Fruits and veggies. It's not just that they have Vitamin C. They have all the right vitamins and lots of phytochemicals for keeping your physiology balanced and protected.

- **Turmeric**

    This unassuming little herb has antibacterial activity. That capability has to help in keeping annoying infections from happening in your nose, throat, and lungs.

- **Amrit**

    Immunity means that you don't get colds. And, as we discussed in Chapter 11, Amrit builds up your immunity.

- **Exercise**

    Exercise may not be so great as a cold remedy. But before you get sick, regular exercise improves circulation and purifies your cells. Pure cells don't get colds.

In fact, as with other ailments in this chapter, all the techniques from this book help to fight colds, flu, and infections; because all strengthen the immune system. If you're having some difficulty with colds despite these gentle recommendations, you can add a little herbal assist to your life—the Bio-Immune tablets that we spoke of in Chapter 9. These puppies build up your immune system. Among the other goals of this synergy of herbs are to get your liver working better (which helps clean out toxins) and to clear out your sinus cavities. As with any defense, it's best to start taking it before you ever need it. Chances are, you'll never know for sure whether you needed it or not. You just won't get a cold.

Juicing Up Your Joints

Joint problems plague many of us. Why should you have to contend with creaky arms and legs? Again, the regimen we speak of here will help avert trouble before it strikes. Turmeric cuts down on inflammation. So does reducing your sugar intake. Green, leafy vegetables fight free radicals, and those marauding free radicals can wreak havoc on your joints. Easy exercise keeps your joints working smoothly without taxing them. As with cancer, you don't want to wait until you have the problem to begin using these preventive measures. If you follow our advice in these pages, you'll help boost your chances of having minimal problems with your joints. That is, you'll never have to say to yourself, "How did I end up with a joint like this?"

Ending Insomnia

Insomnia, if you have it, can be one of the worst of ailments. Little as we seem to value sleep in our society, we begin to cherish it more and more when we are able to get it less and less. Don't sleep at night, and anxiety can rule your day. Colds and infections often seem to get the upper hand. You'd give your kingdom for a good night's sleep.

Practices that normalize your routine help you settle down at night and switch off your mind. Exercise is good. TM relaxes you. Proper diet means that you don't go to bed while your body is wrestling hopelessly to digest something or other. A good routine helps your body attune itself to nature, so that when nature sleeps, you too tend to drift off to the land of nod. Being nice keeps you balanced, and boosts you up with positive neuropeptides.

If you're doing everything we recommend and still find yourself staring at the ceiling at night or getting up to watch *Gilligan's Island* reruns, soothe yourself with the Blissful Sleep tablets we mentioned in Chapter 7. The Indian Valerian and Muskroot in this formulation are natural sleep enhancers. The Winter Cherry helps you resist stress, and it balances the mind and emotions. (A balanced mind, you've probably noticed, has less trouble falling asleep.)

Answering Anxiety

Know one of the worst things about anxiety? It makes you anxious. "Oh, my gosh, I might have another anxiety attack," you think, and, bam, you bring on the attack. Anxiety is so unpleasant that it pretty well takes the shine off of everything else that you do. It's bad for your health, too. According to Vedic medicine, anxiety depletes that substance called ojas, the master coordinator of all the activities in the cell (or, in other words, the whole body). Western medicine has noted a correlation between anxiety and heart attack, though often seeing the anxiety as a symptom of coming trouble rather than a cause.

What helps avert the vexing turn of events known as anxiety? Exercise is good. Meditation helps calm the nerves. Sleep is exceptional, if you can do it. (See preceding section of this chapter.) The phytochemicals in the diet, fighting free radicals, help sidestep emotional upsets. Being nice is a powerful antidote to emotional trouble. All the techniques in this book help.

Need a little something extra to help take the edge off? The herbal formulation known as *Worry-Free* tablets can help you back to normal, and then you can maintain the stability on your own. Here's what's in these tablets:

Herpestis Monniera (true Brahmi), Aloeweed (Shanka-pushpi), Winter Cherry (Ashwagandha), Muskroot (Jatamansi), Pearl Pisti, Greater Galangal, Licorice, Heart-leaved Moonseed (Guduchi).

Some of these herbs are known, traditionally, to smooth out the mind, and these herbs include the Aloeweed, the Brahmi, the Moonseed, and the Muskroot. The Aloeweed and Brahmi nourish your nerve cells, which is a nice antidote to worry. The Moonseed's job is to clear out the microcirculatory channels of the body, including the brain and nerve cells. And the Muskroot, besides settling the mind and emotions, aids natural nerve regeneration.

Take one to two tablets twice a day with warm water or fresh fruit juice. If it's possible, don't take the tablet on an empty stomach, and wait an hour after a full meal. See "Product Recommendations" at the back of the book to find out where to get this.

Take the tablets for a month or so, and you should find that the old, troubling sense of worry just, mysteriously, doesn't trouble you so much any more. Once on an even keel, you'll be able to stay that way just by eating right, sleeping right, and applying a few other modest "anti-cancer" approaches.

Take any sickness—any one at all—and anti-cancer techniques are going to help you against it. If "anti-cancer" isn't your hot button, fine, choose from the list given in this chapter—colds, anxiety, heart disease, creaky joints…You name it; anti-cancer approaches help it.

True, we haven't listed every sickness known to man or woman. There are too many of them, and even medicine doesn't know them all. New ones crop up from time to time. However, this chapter includes quite a list. If you have any one of these problems, your life can be pretty miserable. Maybe you don't have to have the problem before you do something about it. In doing the right thing to prevent cancer, you do the right thing to prevent sickness.

Knowing the wide-ranging health benefits of cancer prevention just may be an incentive to follow the simple recommendations in this book. Sure, you may not be concerned about cancer, but maybe you have a problem with colds, or anxiety, or constipation. Implement "the answer to cancer," and you'll wipe all kinds of other diseases right off your radar screen right along with the long-term risk of cancer.

The "answer to cancer" is the answer to everyday sicknesses and lurking, later sicknesses like heart disease. If you are making yourself healthy from the deepest levels, you're making yourself healthy. Period. You look good. You feel good. You forget all about cancer, colds, or constipation. When you have immunity at work, you don't have to think about sickness. All that is as it should be. After all, there are much better things to think about.

❧ Thirteen

The Secret to "The Answer"

OK, we admit, our title for this book is a little on the brazen side. We speak of "The Answer to Cancer" in a world where the whole medical profession has been throwing up its hands in frustration for decades because it doesn't have anything even beginning to approach an answer.

What's different about us? Cancer, we've explained, happens when cells go berserk. To solve the problem, Western medicine looks at tumors. It looks at cells. It looks at DNA. It looks at the problem itself and perhaps tries to get to its basis, but instead deals with the symptoms.

The Vedic approach also notes that cells have gone berserk. But instead of looking at the tumors, it goes to the basis of everything the cell is doing—namely, the intelligence at the basis of the cell. It goes to the place where the disorder begins, detects irregularities before they turn into cancer, and prevents cancer. That's the secret to our "answer." Why don't we let you in on it a little bit more?

The Secret to Knowing Everything

Instead of starting out with cells, tissue, bones, nosebleeds, x-rays, all the physical stuff, the Vedic approach starts at the level of, well, wholeness, or the unified field from which the universe and the laws of nature originate. This wholeness is consciousness. It starts to know the body by knowing itself. You can't see consciousness. You can't measure it directly with a stethoscope or an x-ray. (X-rays pass right through it.) But it is knowable. And, here's the secret part.—When you get established in the field of pure consciousness, the home of all the laws of nature—a lively field of all possibilities—you have access to knowing everything. The originators of Vedic medicine, and many of their followers throughout the ages, did get established in this field of pure consciousness. (You can, too, but that's not important right now.)

To mainstream Western folks, we acknowledge, the idea of "knowing everything" is outrageous. Let's not mince words about it. To our familiar mindset, you just don't go around claiming the answer to cancer. Western science has a nicely worked out empirical approach where it conducts years of research before it accepts anything as an answer. Solutions to problems (such as the solution of surgery for cancer) build up gradually and painstakingly over time.

Western medicine, logically enough from its perspective, has approached the question of cancer "from the outside in." It has looked at the problem—tumors, basically—and tried ways to fix it. Cut out the tumors. Keep finding better ways to cut them out, like radiation and chemo. Our familiar Western medicine has observed the situation in the human body, and it has tried solutions that it hopes will work. Somebody comes up with an idea, develops a theory, tests the theory in the laboratory, and modifies the theory based on what happens when the theory is put into practice. People keep modifying the theory (making it better), and of course, side effects happen. You take tamoxifen to prevent breast cancer, but it may be a cancer-causer itself.

186

Skeptics will point out that Western medicine has itself begun to explore the possibilities of traditional herbal remedies, diet, daily routine, and lifestyle. However, it feels compelled to explore them in the way we've just mentioned—from the outside in.

The Vedic approach comes at them from all directions—physical, mental, and even spiritual. It doesn't just work from the outside in but, at the same time, from the inside out. It doesn't just respect that intelligence of nature; it becomes the intelligence of nature. It's hard for the Western mind to put concepts to these words. The Vedic approach utilizes consciousness. It dives into it, plays with it, and understands what it does when it does anything. It knows from within itself how intelligence (its very self) unfolds in a plant or how the plant's intelligence influences the body's intelligence. Any intelligence, plant or animal or human, is still intelligence. Western medicine and Vedic medicine may well be converging on the same point as they attempt to solve cancer—namely, that point where intelligence and matter meet in the DNA. As the two approaches converge, though, they take their own routes to get there. Western medicine comes from the outside in. Vedic medicine comes from the outside (physical), from inside (mental), and from way, way inside (spiritual)...that is, from all directions at once.

The Vedic Medicine "Know-it-All"— Bharadwaja

The entire Vedic approach to medicine, according to Vedic tradition, came to light all in one piece. One sage became identical with pure consciousness and, from within himself, saw all of Vedic medicine.—"Here's how to fix this." "Here's how to fix that." You can know everything when you are, yourself, pure consciousness (which is, in fact, everything. If you are everything, you know everything just by knowing yourself).

187

More than 5,000 years ago a sage named *Bharadwaja* lived in an ideal civilization. Things were good. You lived for a really long time. Nobody got sick, and doctors' offices were pretty empty. However, after a very long time without incident, a few people began to develop sniffles, fatigue, little fevers, small worries...signs that things were getting out of sorts. Bharadwaja and other great sages who were also living pure consciousness held a high-level summit and firmly resolved to do something about this terrible disjunction.

Rather than analyzing each sickness and testing each treatment, they collectively settled deep into consciousness. These sages were highly evolved, and a profoundly settled state of awareness developed. In that expanded, probably light-filled state, the sage Bharadwaja cognized the essence of Vedic medicine. It was all there for him. He saw the solutions to disease all at once in perfect form. Traditional Vedic medical practices have been passed on orally ever since. Later on, Bharadwaja's insights were written down in a treatise, which the sage *Charak* then expanded upon. Charak included his interpretations and annotations in this Ayurvedic text known as *Charak Samhita*. This text can be considered the equivalent of a textbook of medicine in modern healthcare systems.

At the risk of introducing a bit too much terminology, we'll mention that Charak's Vedic technology looks for perfect health in these three areas:

- Physical health (which also enjoys a Sanskrit name— *Adhibhautic)*
- Mental health (which, in Sanskrit, is *Adhidaivik)*
- Spiritual health (known in Sanskrit as *Adhyatmik)*

Charak well understood that imbalances in one of these areas would disrupt the others, too. After all, the basis of all three is one and the same thing—consciousness. They're all interconnected. Restoring balance in one restores balance in the others. When you get all three working together in a nice unison, disease just doesn't develop.

Seeing The Body As...Intelligence

How did Bharadwaja see the body? As intelligence. OK, so how do you work on something as rock solid as the body while dealing with something as abstract as "intelligence?" "Intelligence," to the Western mind, just means the mind; the body is "dumb substance." To Vedic medicine, though, the body isn't just something dumb, solid, and separated from intelligence. It actually *is* intelligence. You can influence it with other forms of intelligence—like the intelligence in herbs, the intelligence in the phytochemicals of plants, and your own inner intelligence (which you contact during Transcendental Meditation).

Physical approaches (known in Sanskrit as *Adhibhautic)* define these 5 fundamental elements:

- Space
- Air
- Fire
- Water
- Earth

All of them are forms of intelligence at their basis. The whole approach may seem quaint at first, like some antiquated system of philosophy or something. Or, perhaps you prefer to think of these elements as metaphors. It's not difficult, though, to find examples of each by drawing on Western thinking. Take space, for instance—the body has all kinds of cavities (like the lungs, for one) and gaps like even the tiny synapses between nerves. As for air, the lungs take oxygen from air. They transport it in the blood throughout the body, and the blood is, of course, mostly water. Digestive enzymes produce a digestive "fire" in the belly. We mean, no, your body doesn't burn a hole in itself or anything (but, when you think about it, even that can happen). Earth-like substances? Well, the bones are a good start.

What do these five elements have to do with intelligence? If you peek a bit into any ingredient of the body, pretty soon

189

you get to "empty space." And that empty space isn't just nothing. It's empty space with a particular character. It's consciousness. Consider how physics analyzes matter, and you can look at the body in the same way. Any element consists of molecules. At the basis of molecules are atoms. At the basis of atoms are what physics refers to as quantum particles, which are already part matter and part energy. (That is, these quantum particles are that level of life where matter and energy are merely different aspects of the same thing.) Beyond those particles is the level of pure energy...which, ta da, is also pure intelligence.

What, exactly, is that intelligence, and what makes it different from just, plain nothing? It is "laws." The laws of nature that govern the activity of the element reside at that level of pure intelligence. Technically, all the laws are there all the time. But those laws make an organ work properly. The intelligence of a liver cell continuously directs it in its activity as a liver cell (and not as a lung cell, skin cell, or cancer cell). The organ expresses its own inner intelligence. Likewise every cell and every complete human body expresses the intelligence within it.

If we are not in the habit of thinking of the body itself as intelligence, we certainly aren't accustomed to thinking of a single cell in that way. A cell is just a shape under a microscope. Each cell, though, is an organism just like the full-sized body. A cell has a brain (the DNA). It has its own organs (called organelles) that carry out different functions. The cell even has a skeleton, made up of microtubules. And the skin of the cell is the membrane that holds it together.

When you begin to look at what a cell does, you can see its intelligence working. On the surface of the cell are pores and other types of gateways. These gateways, in some cases, are selective. That is, they apply intelligence as they allow only certain types of molecules to pass through or as they respond in special ways to other molecules such as neurotransmitters. (Neurotransmitters are chemical substances that transmit information.) The selective gateways, called receptors, respond and interact using transmitters. They interact with the "brain" of the cell—that very DNA that has to stay intact to protect against disease or even cancer.

When a cell stays intelligent, it's healthy. When it loses intelligence, watch out. That's when trouble is sure to come up. The *Adhibhautic* approach, for its part, works on the intelligence of the cell to keep that trouble from arising.

The Mind? Intelligence, Too

How did Bharadwaja see the mind? Also as intelligence. If you say "mind" to someone familiar with only the Western approach, the person right away tends to picture something like psychoanalysis or psychological counseling. Everybody has heard of psychosomatic illness, and everybody knows vaguely that there is some connection between the health of the mind and overall health.

But the Western approach isn't particularly systematic and mechanical in working with the mind, and it tends to get stuck in detours and blind alleys. Working "from the outside in" to analyze a single dream could lead to endless related associations. (The whole process might not even get you very far.)

Vedic medicine, which thinks of the mind as intelligence to begin with, does all kinds of mechanical things to influence intelligence. The mind, according to the Vedic approach, has intelligence flowing through it just as do the body and the cell. The intelligence is both abstract and concrete. That is, it is both intelligence itself and intelligence expressed through various chemicals, enzymes, and other substances. Traditional Ayurveda knows that intelligence and influences it to strengthen the mind, including that mind of the cell (the DNA).

You can sip some tea and influence the mind. Be nice to somebody and make yourself healthy. Settle into a cozy, transcendental frame of mind, and enrich your level of happiness. Take a walk, and change your whole mental outlook. When

191

Charak saw everything all at once on the level of consciousness, he saw the nature of mind as intelligence, and he saw
how to sweeten the mind in various ways.

Science, it's true, has begun to come closer and closer to
seeing the body as intelligence itself. Science has found that
the limbic area of the brain surrounds the hypothalamus at the
center of the brain and correlates with deep emotional states.
The hypothalamus is the "brain's brain"—the central switchboard of the body. The hypothalamus puts its smartness to
work all the time as it regulates body temperature, thirst,
hunger, blood sugar and—to mention a few more things—
growth, sleeping, waking, and emotions.

The West is beginning to acknowledge that when the brain
works, it does so in a mechanical way. The limbic area of the
brain stimulates the hypothalamus to release neuropeptides
(substances that convey information). These neuropeptides
stimulate the pituitary gland to release certain hormones, and
from the hormones arises activity in the thyroid and the adrenal glands. "Adrenaline" from the adrenal glands is familiar to
everybody. Secrete some, and you get angry or otherwise
supercharged. The point is that Western medicine recognizes
that tiny substances moving around in the body cause all kinds
of things to happen—the emotions and other activities we
experience every day. Intelligence is at work.

Vedic medicine has always worked on the mechanical level
of the mind's intelligence. It doesn't get caught up in psychoanalysis. Vedic science knows specific indications of a mind
that is strong, weak, or unbalanced. It knows what those various states of mind are likely to mean for health.

The Vedic texts are pretty detailed. When Charak wrote
down Bharadwaja's perceptions, he had his work cut out for
him. For instance, Charak talks about five mental approaches
for mind. (As we said earlier, the Sanskrit name for approaches
to health on the level of the mind is *Adhidaivik.*) Here are
Charak's five mental approaches, with the Sanskrit names in
parentheses, just for the fun of it:

1. Transcendence *(Samadhi)*—Transcendence is good. It's an expanded state of the mind. You transcend during Transcendental Meditation. Transcending creates balance in your mind and in the all-important body, too. During transcending, you merge with your higher Self.

2. Memory *(Smriti)*—This memory doesn't mean just remembering where you put your car keys. It's the memory of the unity of life—knowing that the transcendence is what you are. The effect of this kind of memory is pretty cool.—Fearlessness.

3. Patience *(Dhairya)*—Some experts translate this mental approach as "courage." The two go together anyway—courage and patience. When you have total knowledge of life, you can patiently wait and watch things unfold. And you have no fear about the outcome.

4. Knowledge *(Gyan)*—You do learn things from books, movies, TV, and walking around the streets. That kind of knowledge is "Gyan," which comes in handy in life.

5. Wisdom *(Vigyan)*—You can tell from the name that this knowledge has something to do with the one just above it. When you have an experience, you begin to make proper sense out of the knowledge you have learned from books and places. In turn, you gain wisdom.

When the mind is working right, all five of these mental approaches are strong. By looking at the categories, you can begin to sense that having a strong mind would make you strong in lots of good ways. When the mind isn't working right, it's a whole different story.

When the mind is pure, then it lives all five of these qualities fully. The same is true for a cell. When the cell loses touch with its inner intelligence, it can behave weirdly. In our terms, it can become cancerous. Western medicine really hasn't been equipped for working with the cell to keep it in tune with its own intelligence, so that it stays on track. Vedic medicine is equipped for that.

The Spirit? Nothing But Intelligence

How does Bharadwaja see the spirit? Also as intelligence. In the West, traditionally, we do see the spirit as something abstract, even as a form of intelligence. But there is all kinds of confusion about dealing with the spirit, and Western approaches are hardly as mechanical and simple as the Vedic approaches.

What is the spirit in the West? Explanations are all over the map. It's "abstract soul" (which, of course, you couldn't massage with an herbalized oil). It's something ephemeral. It's energy. It's the soul. It's...hard to say. Vedic medicine, though, takes the spirit head on. Vedic technologies for spiritual health, contained in the Charak's *Adhyatmik* approach clear the way for the spirit to shine through without obstructions.

The heart of Vedic spiritual technology is a simple understanding, expressed in the Sanskrit phrase *"swashmin tishthati iti swasthya,"* which translates as "the person who remains in the Self all the time is healthy." That is, if you could only remain fully open to the spirit all the time, then you wouldn't crave alcohol, cigarettes, fatty foods, sugar, or any of the other carcinogens. Remain in the Self all the time, through all that you do, and you remain healthy.

The term used to define health in Sanskrit is *Swastha.* "Swa" means "Self" and "astha" means "established." According to the Vedic tradition, "one who is established in the Self is healthy, established in the area where all the laws of nature reside."

A well-known Vedic proverb says, *"brahma bhavati sarati,"* which translates as "For those established in self-referral consciousness, the infinite organizing power of the creator becomes the charioteer of all actions." When you surrender to the abstract universal Self and are established in your own being, then the universal Self becomes the charioteer of your life.

In the Vedic texts, the "chariot" has a special metaphysical meaning. It refers to the physiology. The chariot stands on the battlefield of life as a vehicle for the natural process of evolution. Yoked to the chariot, in the classic Vedic picture, are 10 horses. Five are the sense organs, and five are the organs of action (the mouth for speech; the hands and legs for movement; the organs of elimination; and the organs of procreation). The yoked horses are white, the color symbolizing purity. Two passengers are in the chariot—the small self (the ego), and the large Self (*Atma* or soul). The reins are the mind.

In the ordinary scheme of things for the human, without Vedic technologies, the horses aren't pure. They're a bit wild. The small self is at their mercy. Most of us are quite familiar with the situation facing the bewildered small self. People don't eat right, don't sleep right, and don't behave right. Cravings dominate. People unintentionally violate laws of nature, and their health suffers. The conditions that lead to cancer are free to flourish.

Vedic technologies can install white horses and hand the reins over to the larger Self. To leave behind the metaphor for a moment, we can say that you can set up the conditions where you spontaneously guide the sense organs and organs of action in the proper direction. Operating from your own inner Self, you spontaneously do what is best for your body.

Just as for mind and body, you need to apply technologies if you want to put the Self in charge. You can't simply decide to remain in the Self and have it happen. The Self is too abstract. Meditation is a technology to open individual awareness to the abstract Self, but all the other things we've talked about help as well—sleep, turmeric, phytochemicals, everything. You may not think of eating cooked squash as a way to calm the spirit, but Vedic medicine does, and it knows why it works.

Granting Yourself A Little Immunity

So, can the knowledge of Bharadwaja and Charak get us to the highest ideal of prevention—namely, to full immunity? Yes, actually, you can get the intelligence of mind, body, and spirit to work collectively to create strong immunity (which seems like an awfully bold pronouncement when talking of cancer). If your immune system is faulty, you can get cancer. If your immune system is strong, even super strong, you don't get cancer. For immunity—as for mind, body, and spirit—intelligence is the basis of all the rest that is going on. Vedic technologies work with that intelligence.

The name for immunity in Sanskrit is *Bala.*

Bala can be of three kinds (Sanskrit in parentheses):

- Innate *(Sahaj)*
- According to time, season, and age *(Kalaj)*
- Acquired *(Yuktikrit)*

Sahaj, or innate immunity, comes by birth and derives from the physical and mental strength of the mother and father. Western medicine recognizes that heredity plays a role in whether or not a person gets cancer. If immunity is inborn, you can't really change it. Knowing your degree of innate immunity can help in determining whether or not you are susceptible to certain forms of cancer.

You can strengthen Kalaj immunity (the immunity according to time, season, and age). Certain foods are better at certain times of the year. Certain behaviors are better at certain times of life. In the winter when it's cold, eat hot foods. In the summer when it's hot, eat cool foods. Some easy guidelines can help you maintain your Kalaj immunity. Also, there are Vedic preparations and behavioral *rasayanas* to strengthen your Kalaj immunity.

Of all three of these immunities, acquired immunity probably seems to offer the most possibilities to the Western reader. According to Vedic technology, those with low or weak immunity can develop strong immunity. The same techniques discussed in this book for fostering prevention also culture acquired immunity—diet, behaviors, rasayanas (both herbal remedies and behaviors), massage therapies, and so on. People can acquire immunity, and they can acquire immunity even with regard to the killer itself—cancer.

A Sanskrit phrase describes how rasayanas work to develop immunity. *"Labhopayohi sashtanam rasadinam rasayanam."* A translation for the phrase might go like this: "Excellence of the principles supporting the body tissues can create a strong immune system, and Vedic technologies (rasayanas) strengthen those principles that support the body tissues." (Note where the solution comes from—from inside. Principles create strength. And principles come from consciousness.)

Strengthened immunity also has a powerful benefit for those with cancer who are undergoing treatment. Chemotherapy has known, regrettable toxicity of its own. Those undergoing chemotherapy suffer depression, nausea, and various other unpleasant effects. Strengthening immunity with Vedic technologies also strengthens immunity against poisoning from your own chemotherapy. It counteracts the negative effects of the chemotherapy, as we discussed in Chapter 11.

Putting a Priority on Prevention

Working on the level of inner intelligence (instead of on the level of disease) has an interesting result for the Vedic approach. For a Western doctor to treat you, you have to be sick. For an Ayurvedic doctor (Vaidya), the sickness isn't a prerequisite. You can see a Vaidya no matter how good you feel, and he can probably help you feel a little better. The name for what the Vaidya does is "prevention."

Think about it for a moment. If you feel that something may be wrong, perhaps even that cancer could be developing, you don't have much luck with contemporary Western medicine unless something actually is drastically wrong. Typically, if you go to a Western physician, the well-intentioned health provider conducts tests such as the PSA test for prostate cancer or a mammogram for possible breast cancer. If the tests don't detect actual cancer, you get a smile and the words "Come back when you have problems."

Vedic medicine takes the opposite approach. "Regardless of how you feel, let me examine you for possible imbalances. Let me see how well the intelligence is working in your mind, body, and spirit. If you have imbalances, then, yes, you have the basis for disease, even if you don't actually have full-blown cancer."

If you have imbalances, you have ama in the system—the end-product of poorly digested food. As we discussed in Chapter 2, ama is toxic material and creates imbalance in the body. No one has yet clearly spelled out the equivalent to ama in Western medicine, but Western medicine does know that circulating toxins usually begin in the digestive system, where ama also begins. Ayurveda can detect and counteract ama.

Vedic technology also knows and understands another substance we talked about in Chapter 2, an immune enhancer created by perfect digestion. This substance, ojas, is nothing less than the very substance that connects consciousness with matter. If Western medicine (coming from the outside in) and Vedic medicine (coming from the inside out) were to meet at one point, that point would be ojas. It is a substance. As a substance, according to Vedic texts, ojas is white and oily. It pervades the body.

It is also consciousness. It is, you might say, liquid consciousness. Ojas is the "lamp at the door" between consciousness and matter. According to Vedic medicine, it literally helps consciousness slide into matter. If it flows freely throughout the body, then intelligence remains maximum throughout the body.

If there are blockages in the body due to ama, then the intelligence cannot flow freely. Physiological disorders and diseases arise. Cancer can arise. By eliminating ama and strengthening ojas, you can create the free flow of intelligence throughout your body. Cancer would not arise.

If you could create a body that was nothing but pure consciousness, cancer would not be a possibility. Even by moving in the direction of such a healthy body, you increase cell intelligence and minimize the chances of disease.

A simple Sanskrit proverb, a phrase from the Vedas, is *"Heyam dukham anagatam,"* which translates as "Avert the danger which has not yet come." This angle is the essence of all Vedic technology.—Treat disease if you must, but, above all, prevent it if you can. Prevention. Prevention. Prevention.

Rather than looking at disease, Vedic technology looks at health. "What is the ultimate definition of health?" it asks, and the response is "fully developed mind, body, and spirit." What is the indicator of fully perfect health? Ojas. What is the indicator of imbalance? Ama. For any disease, such as cancer, Vedic technology says you should know the cause of the disease with respect to ideal health. The cause will be some form of imbalance. You then work on the level of the intelligence of the body to restore the balance, and Vedic technologies know how to do that very well.

Evening Out the "Environment"

While we're talking about the comprehensive Vedic approaches, we'd be remiss if we didn't mention another pretty big influence on your health—the environment. Other things can come into play for cancer prevention than what you eat or even the condition of your spirit. Your environment can be a factor, both near environment and far. Your house can be a factor, and we're not just talking about radon. The shape of the house and the placement of the rooms matters, according to Vedic understanding. Far environment? The planets. They may seem too far away to have any effect, but Vedic tradition understands their effect quite intimately.

First, consider your house (or apartment, cottage, condo, houseboat, igloo, tepee, you name it). Your house affects your physiology. Here's another, brief Sanskrit term for you from the ancient literature—*Vastu*. Vastu refers to the design and structure of a building and its harmony with natural law. If a building has proper Vastu, it helps keep you healthy. If it doesn't have proper Vastu, it doesn't help keep you healthy (and can even make you sick).

199

To understand how the Vedic tradition views Vastu, think about the human body. In the body, the organs are supposed to be in certain specific places, not others. The human heart, that much valued organ, has to be in its special place—namely, in the center (or, as the old saying goes, at the heart of things). From its central position it distributes life-giving blood throughout your body. The heart, inside the breastbone, is protected, and free from obstructions. Likewise, the center of your house should be free from obstructions and open in all directions. Most houses aren't that way today, we readily concede. But it's best for health when they are like that. They don't have to be wide open to the outside air. That can be cold in winter. But they should be open to the sun. For example, the main entrance to the house should be on the east wall. This means the house is facing the vibrant, life-giving rays of the rising sun each morning and gains the full benefit of being bathed, head on, in those rays.

According to Vastu, each room of the house should be in a specific place, just as each organ is in a specific place within the body. What happens if the rooms aren't in the right places? The body, again, is an instructive example. There can be examples in the body where organs, or parts of organs, are not in their proper places. Sometimes, due to congenital defect, the gastric mucosa (stomach lining) may be present in an abnormal place, like the small bowel. That's not good. When it does its work from there instead of from inside the stomach, it causes disturbances, such as an ulcer. Likewise, activities that occur in the various rooms of the house may run into difficulties if the rooms are not in their proper place. They will not receive the full support of nature that would otherwise occur. The end result of this may be various problems in life, including illness.

The house is one environment we tend to occupy at least some of the time. Whether you're inside the house or not, you occupy other environments—the solar system, the galaxy, the universe. All these things have an influence, and Vedic tradition understands that influence and can work with it to possibly avert calamities like cancer. Each person—during each period of the day, month, or year—is immersed in the influences of different planets. Sometimes one planet has stronger influence, sometimes another; and that affects how a person feels. Vedic technologies, using a mathematical approach called *Jyotish* (Vedic astrology—not to be confused with the Western type of astrology) can identify a person's risk of certain diseases. This science looks at a person's exact date, time, and place of birth and, from there, calculates the planetary influences.

Good old Mars, for instance, often so visible in the night sky, brings an aggressive influence. If a person has a strong influence of Mars at a particular time, he or she may be a bit quarrelsome. Conflicts may lead to problems and stress. What does Vedic tradition recommend that one do about it? It offers technologies called *Yagyas* that use special vibratory techniques (mantras) to diffuse the problems coming from planetary influences.

Some quite practical techniques arise from knowing about the environmental influences on the physiology. Here's one simple recommendation we can make here. Sleep with your head to the East (the headboard of your bed would be against the east wall of your bedroom). It makes a difference. Sleeping with your head to the East brings the most balance to you as you sleep. Sleeping with your head to the North has the most harmful effect. Here's why. Your nervous system, brain, and spinal cord act as an electromagnetic field. Your nerves are transmission lines, literally. Wherever there is electricity, as there is in the body, there is magnetism. The earth, too, has its magnetic field. The North Pole is, of course, the North Pole of the earth. The head is the North Pole of the body. Line them up in the same direction, and they repel each other. That's not good. Sleep with the head to the East, though, and that is good. This is supported by research conducted by Rajeswari and Associates.

The healthier your environment, the stronger your protection against cancer. And your environment, in the Vedic tradition, includes everything around you, near and far—your workplace, your house, your neighborhood, and on and on to the planets and the stars.

Conclusion

Cancer isn't really so hard, then…not if you go at it from all sides the way the Vedic tradition allows. You can fix cancer by never letting it happen. That may sound good in theory, but how do you actually go about something like "enlivening the intelligence of your own cells?" You'd have a good deal of difficulty just working on your own to do it. You wouldn't know what to eat, what routine to follow, what to avoid. Anyone would have trouble evolving a complete theory of how to wake up the intelligence of mind, body, and spirit. You can't just pop a lot of Vitamin C or add tons of turmeric or garlic to your foods and expect to develop cancer immunity.

Even meditating, arguably the most powerful of the technologies in this book, might not be enough by itself to prevent cancer. Cells that are going a little bit astray need some gentle coaxing, from the right neuropeptides or carefully chosen phytochemicals.

How do you know how to coax them in the right way? You could call a summit meeting of enlightened sages the way Bharadwaja did. That works, if you're completely at one with the level of pure consciousness yourself. Or, you could apply techniques passed on from Bharadwaja's time, techniques that work on the level of the consciousness of the cell. Those techniques are the techniques in this book.

Apply these techniques, and you're doing the best things you can to protect against ever getting cancer. The techniques work from the level of consciousness, but they work on all levels of the mind, body, and spirit. They prevent cells from going berserk. The Vedic tradition has taught them to us, and we're passing them along to you.

And now you know our secret.

❧ Selected References

BOOKS

A Six Month Course in Yoga Asanas. SRM International Publications, undated.

American Heart Association and American Cancer Society. *Living Well, Staying Well: The Ultimate Guide to Help Prevent Heart Disease and Cancer.* New York:Times Books, 1996.

Boik, J. *Cancer & Natural Medicine: A Textbook of Basic Science and Clinical Research.* Princeton, Minn.: Oregon Medical Press, 1996.

Cancer Facts & Figures 2002. Atlanta: American Cancer Society, Inc., 2002.

Cancer Prevention & Early Detection: Facts & Figures 2002. Atlanta:American Cancer Society, Inc., 2002.

Lamb, J. F., C. G. Ingram, I. A. Johnston, R. M. Pitman. *Essentials of Physiology.* Oxford: Blackwell Scientific Publications, 1991.

Mowrey, D. B. *Next Generation Herbal Medicine: Guaranteed Potency Herbs.* New Canaan, Conn.: Keats Publishing, Inc., 1990.

Murray, M.T., J. E. Pizzorno. *Encyclopedia of Natural Medicine.* Rocklin, Calif.: Prima Publishing, 1991.

Newmark,T. M., P. Schulick. *Beyond Aspirin: Nature's Answer to Arthritis, Cancer, & Alzheimer's Disease.* Prescott,Ariz.: Hohm Press, 2000.

Pawlak, L. *A Perfect 10: Phyto "New-trients" Against Cancers.* Emeryville, Calif.: Biomed General Corp., 1998.

Pert, C. B. *Molecules of Emotion.* New York:Touchstone (Simon & Schuster), 1999.

Sharma, H. *Freedom from Disease: How to Control Free Radicals, A Major Cause of Aging and Disease.* Toronto: Veda Publishing, 1993.

———. *Awakening Nature's Healing Intelligence.* Twin Lakes,Wis.: Lotus Press, 1997.

Sharma, H., C. Clark. *Contemporary Ayurveda.* London: Churchill Livingstone, 1998.

Sharma, R.K., B. Dash, trans. *Charaka Samhita.* Varanasi, India: Chowkhamba Sanskrit Series Office, 1977.

Walters, R. *Options: The Alternative Cancer Therapy Book.* Garden City Park, N.Y.: Avery Publishing Group Inc., 1993.

Wiley, T.S., B. Formby. *Lights Out: Sleep, Sugar, and Survival.* New York: Pocket Books (Simon and Schuster), 2000.

ARTICLES

Blaylock, R. L. A review of conventional cancer prevention and treatment and the adjunctive use of nutraceutical supplements and antioxidants: Is there a danger or a significant benefit? *Journal of the American Nutraceutical Association* 2000;3(3): 17–35.

Bravo, L. Polyphenols: Chemistry, dietary sources, metabolism, and nutritional significance. *Nutrition Reviews* 1998; 56(11):317–333.

Bristol, J.B. Colorectal cancer and diet: A case-control study with special reference to dietary fibre and sugar. *Proceedings of the American Association of Cancer Research* March 1985;26:206.

Campbell, J. D. Cancer prevention. *Townsend Letter for Doctors* November 1994;136:1225.

Dileepan, K. N., V. Patel, H. M. Sharma, D. J. Stechschulte. Priming of splenic lymphocytes after ingestion of an Ayurvedic herbal food supplement: Evidence for an immunomodulatory effect. *Biochemical Archives* 1990;6:267–274.

Dileepan, K.N., S. T. Varghese, J. C. Page, D. J. Stechschulte. Enhanced lymphoproliferative response, macrophage mediated tumor cell killing and nitric oxide production after ingestion of an Ayurvedic drug. *Biochemical Archives* 1993;9:365–374.

Dogra, J., A. Bhargava (SPON: H. Sharma). Lipid peroxide in ischemic heart disease (IHD): Inhibition by Maharishi Amrit Kalash (MAK-4 and MAK-5) herbal mixtures. *Federation of*

American Societies for Experimental Biology Journal 2000;14(4):A121 (Abstract).

Dogra, J., N. Grover, P. Kumar, N. Aneja. Indigenous free radical scavenger MAK 4 and 5 in angina pectoris: Is it only a placebo? *Journal of the Association of Physicians of India* 1994;42(6):466–467.

Engineer, F. N., H. M. Sharma, C. Dwivedi. Protective effects of M-4 and M-5 on Adriamycin-induced microsomal lipid peroxidation and mortality. *Biochemical Archives* 1992; 8:267–272.

Fukuda, Y., M. Nagata, T. Osawa, M. Namiki. Contribution of lignan analogues to antioxidative activity of refined unroasted sesame seed oil. *Journal of the American Oil Chemists' Society* 1986;63(8):1027–1031.

Huang, M. T., T. Lysz, T. Ferraro, A. H. Conney. Inhibitory effects of curcumin on tumor promotion and arachidonic acid metabolism in mouse epidermis. In: L. Wattenberg, M. Lipkin, C. W. Boone, G. J. Kelloff, eds. *Cancer Chemoprevention.* Boca Raton, Fla.: CRC Press, Inc., 1992:375–391.

Inaba, R., H. Sugiura, H. Iwata. Immunomodulatory effects of Maharishi Amrit Kalash 4 and 5 in mice. *Japanese Journal of Hygiene* 1995;50(4):901–905.

Inaba, R., H. Sugiura, H. Iwata, H. Mori, T. Tanaka. Immunomodulation by Maharishi Amrit Kalash 4 in mice. *Journal of Applied Nutrition* 1996;48(1/2):10–21.

Inaba R., H. Sugiura, H. Iwata, T. Tanaka. Dose-dependent activation of immune function in mice by ingestion of Maharishi Amrit Kalash 5. *Environmental Health and Preventive Medicine* 1997;2(1):35–39.

Lee, J. Y., A. N. Hanna, J. A. Lott, H. M. Sharma. The antioxidant and antiatherogenic effects of MAK-4 in WHHL rabbits. *Journal of Alternative and Complementary Medicine* 1996;2(4): 463–478.

Mazzoleni, G., W. L. W. Hsiao, M. Statuto, F. Ferrari, M. Marra, H. Sharma, D. Di Lorenzo. Anti-tumor effects of the antioxidant natural products Maharishi Amrit Kalash-4 and -5 (MAK) on cell transformation *in vitro* and in liver carcinogenesis in mice. *Journal of Applied Nutrition* 2002;52(2/3):45-63.

Misra, N. C., H. M. Sharma, A. Chaturvedi, Ramakant, S. Srivastav, V. Devi, P. Kakkar, Vishwanathan, S. M. Natu, J. Bogra. Antioxidant adjuvant therapy using a natural herbal mixture (MAK) during intensive chemotherapy: Reduction in toxicity. A prospective study of 62 patients. In: R. S. Rao, M. G. Deo, L. D. Sanghvi, eds. *Proceedings of the XVI International Cancer Congress.* Bologna, Italy: Monduzzi Editore, 1994:3099-3102.

Nagabhushan, M., S. V. Bhide. Nonmutagenicity of curcumin and its antimutagenic action versus chili and capsaicin. *Nutrition and Cancer* 1986;8(3):201-210.

Orme-Johnson, D. W. Medical care utilization and the Transcendental Meditation program. *Psychosomatic Medicine* 1987;49:493-507.

Patel, V. K., J. Wang, R. N. Shen, H. M. Sharma, Z. Brahmi. Reduction of metastases of Lewis Lung Carcinoma by an Ayurvedic food supplement in mice. *Nutrition Research* 1992;12:51-61.

Peters, J. M., S. Preston-Martin, S. J. London, J. D. Bowman, J. D. Buckley, D. C. Thomas. Processed meats and risk of childhood leukemia (California, USA). *Cancer Causes and Control* 1994;5:195-202.

Phillips, R. L. Role of life-style and dietary habits in risk of cancer among Seventh-Day Adventists. *Cancer Research* 1975;35:3513-3522.

Phytochemicals for cancer protection. *American Institute for Cancer Research NEWSLETTER,* Winter 1995, Issue 46.

Pienta, K. J., D. S. Coffey. Cellular harmonic information transfer through a tissue tensegrity-matrix system. *Medical Hypotheses* 1991;34:88-95.

Polasa, K., B. Sesikaran, T. P. Krishna, K. Krishnaswamy. Turmeric (*Curcuma longa*)-induced reduction in urinary mutagens. *Food and Chemical Toxicology* 1991;29(10):699-706.

Prasad, K. N. , J. Edwards-Prasad, S. Kentroti, C. Brodie, A. Vernadakis. Ayurvedic (Science of Life) agents induce differentiation in murine neuroblastoma cells in culture. *Neuropharmacology* 1992;31(6):599-607.

Prasad, M. L., P. Parry, C. Chan. Ayurvedic agents produce differential effects on murine and human melanoma cells *in vitro. Nutrition and Cancer* 1993;20(1):79-86.

Pratt, R. R. The new interface between music and medicine. In: R. Spintge, R. Droh, eds. *MusicMedicine.* St. Louis, Mo.: MMB Music, Inc., 1992:6-18.

Rajeswari, K. R., M. Satyanarayana, P. V. Sanker Narayan, S. Subrahmanyam. Effect of extremely low frequency magnetic field on serum cholinesterase in humans and animals. *Indian Journal of Experimental Biology* 1985;23: 194-197.

Reddy, A. Ch. P., B. R. Lokesh. Studies on spice principles as antioxidants in the inhibition of lipid peroxidation of rat liver microsomes. *Molecular and Cellular Biochemistry* 1992; 111:117-124.

Salerno, J. W., D. E. Smith. The use of sesame oil and other vegetable oils in the inhibition of human colon cancer growth in vitro. *Anticancer Research* 1991;11:209-216.

Sarasua, S., D. A. Savitz. Cured and broiled meat consumption in relation to childhood cancer: Denver, Colo. (United States). *Cancer Causes and Control* 1994;5:141-148.

Schardt, D. Phytochemicals: Plants against cancer. *Nutrition Action Health Letter* April 1994;21(3):9-11.

Shalini, V. K., L. Srinivas. Lipid peroxide induced DNA damage: Protection by turmeric *(Curcuma longa). Molecular and Cellular Biochemistry* 1987;77:3-10.

Sharma, H., J. Guenther, A. Abu-Ghazaleh, C. Dwivedi. Effects of Ayurvedic food supplement M-4 on cisplatin-induced changes in glutathione and glutathione-S-transferase activity. In: R. S. Rao, M. G. Deo, L. D. Sanghvi, eds. *Proceedings of the XVI International Cancer Congress.* Bologna, Italy: Monduzzi Editore, 1994:589-592.

Sharma, H. M., Free radicals and natural antioxidants in health and disease. *Journal of Applied Nutrition* 2002;52(2/3): 26–44.

Sharma, H. M., C. N. Alexander. Maharishi Ayurveda: Research review. Part 2: Maharishi Ayurveda herbal food supplements and additional strategies. *Complementary Medicine International* 1996;3(2):17–28.

Sharma, H. M., C. Dwivedi, B. C. Satter, H. Abou-Issa. Antineoplastic properties of Maharishi Amrit Kalash, an Ayurvedic food supplement, against 7,12 Dimethylbenz(a) anthracene-induced mammary tumors in rats. *Journal of Research and Education in Indian Medicine* 1991;10(3): 1–8.

Sharma, H. M., C. Dwivedi, B. C. Satter, K. P. Gudehithlu, H. Abou-Issa, W. Malarkey, G. A. Tejwani. Antineoplastic properties of Maharishi-4 against DMBA-induced mammary tumors in rats. *Pharmacology Biochemistry & Behavior* 1990;35: 767–773.

Sharma, H. M., A. N. Hanna, E. M. Kauffman, H. A. I. Newman. Inhibition of human low-density lipoprotein oxidation in vitro by Maharishi Ayur-Veda herbal mixtures. *Pharmacology Biochemistry and Behavior* 1992;43:1175–1182.

Sharma, H. M., E. M. Kauffman, R. E. Stephens. Effect of different sounds on growth of human cancer cell lines in vitro. *Alternative Therapies in Clinical Practice* 1996;3(4):25–32.

Smith, D. E., J. W. Salerno. Selective growth inhibition of a human malignant melanoma cell line by sesame oil in vitro. *Prostaglandins Leukotrienes and Essential Fatty Acids* 1992;46:145–150.

Srinivas, L., V. K. Shalini. DNA damage by smoke: Protection by turmeric and other inhibitors of ROS. *Free Radical Biology and Medicine* 1991;11:277–283.

Srivastava, A., A. Samaiya, V. Taranikanti, P. Kachroo, O. H. Coshic, R. Parshad, V. Seenu, S. Chumber, M. C. Misra, H. Sharma. Maharishi Amrit Kalash (MAK) reduces chemotherapy toxicity in breast cancer patients. *Federation of American Societies for Experimental Biology Journal* 2000;14(4): A720 (Abstract).

Stevens, M. M. The effects of a sesame oil mouthrinse on the number of oral bacteria colony types. Presented at the 11th International Symposium on Dental Hygiene, Ottawa, Canada, June 1989.

Sugano, M., T. Inoue, K. Koba. Influence of sesame lignans on various lipid parameters in rats. *Agricultural and Biological Chemistry* 1990;54(10):2669–2673.

Sundaram, V., A. N. Hanna, G. P. Lubow, L. Koneru, J. M. Falko, H. M. Sharma. Inhibition of low-density lipoprotein oxidation by oral herbal mixtures Maharishi Amrit Kalash-4 and Maharishi Amrit Kalash-5 in hyperlipidemic patients. *American Journal of Medical Sciences* 1997;314(5): 303–310.

Thill, J. Reducing the toxic effects of chemotherapy: New research reports a significant decrease in chemo toxicity with a natural, Ayurvedic herbal formula. *Townsend Letter for Doctors & Patients* August/September 2000:134–138.

Thom, J. A., J. E. Morris, A. Bishop, N. J. Blacklock. The influence of refined carbohydrate on urinary calcium excretion. *British Journal of Urology* 1978;50(7):459–464.

Triguna, B. D. Concept of rasayana in Ayurveda. First Conference on Ayurveda, Bharatiya Vidya Bhavan, New York, Oct. 31–Nov. 1, 1998.

WEBSITES

American Cancer Society, http://www.cancer.org
American Institute for Cancer Research, http://www.aicr.org
Maharishi Ayurveda Products International, http://www.mapi. com
National Cancer Institute, http://www.nci.nih.gov
Transcendental Meditation, http://www.tm.org
UC Davis Health System, http://healthtip.ucdavis.edu/aosshb. html

Resource for Ayurveda: http://www.avertcancer.com

❧ Product Recommendations

This book is all about making your body into a do-it-yourself anti-cancer machine. If you eat right, sleep right, and be nice to people (along with a few other things), your body gets too strong to ever have its cells fall into confusion and disarray. Sometimes, though, a human system may have fallen into some unfavorable tendencies that are just hard to reverse. The body can use a little boost from somewhere, such as from gentle little herbs, fruits, and other plants you can find in nature. The ingredients can reach their fullest potential (and help your body reach its) when combined with each other in the right proportions in the right ways. Ayurveda has the knowledge of how to properly do this.

We've made a few recommendations in the course of this book to help your body reach its best anti-cancer equilibrium. Here are the herbal supplements we've recommended:

Amrit Ambrosia Tablets—These tablets are focused free radical devourers.

Amrit Nectar Paste—This fruit concentrate has lots of anti-cancer properties.

Amrit Nectar Tablets—Chemotherapy patients may have trouble eating the Amrit Nectar paste. These tablets have all the power of the fruit concentrate, but they don't have the honey and sugar. Oh, and they don't have ghee (clarified butter) either.

Be Trim Tea—If you're addicted to sugar, you can really crave the sweet stuff. Take some of this tea, and the craving is supposed to drop right down to just about nothing.

Bio-Immune Tablets—This is not an antibiotic, but it is heck on bacteria. These tablets have zinc, mica, and pearl and take six months to make. They help your liver and your blood and make it easier for your cells to communicate with each other.

Blissful Sleep Tablets—Despite your best intentions, sometimes you just don't sleep so well. These natural supplements just may quiet you down and get you over the hump into a good night's sleep.

Elim-Tox-O Tablets—Exercise will help clean out your cells pretty nicely. As an added boost, this phytochemical mixture helps purify your liver, metabolism, and perspiration.

Herbal Digest Tablets—Sometimes, even if you're eating right, you're not really getting all the benefits of the nutrients from your food. This is due to improper digestion. You can perk up your digestion a tad with these tablets.

Worry-Free Tablets—The heart-leaved Moonseed (Guduchi) in these tablets will help clean out your microcirculatory channels. That's refreshing. Other ingredients settle your mind and emotions and, besides, help you sleep.

Youthful Skin Oil—Sesame oil is good, but some people who have sensitive skin use the Youthful Skin oil instead. It contains Jojoba oil, Almond oil, and other soothing ingredients along with the Sesame oil.

You can order them all from the same source—Maharishi Ayurveda Products International, Inc. (MAPI). Here's the contact information:

MAPI
1068 Elkton Drive
Colorado Springs, CO 80907
Phone: 800-255-8332
Fax: 719-536-4003
Email: info@mapi.com
Web address: www.mapi.com

❧ Index